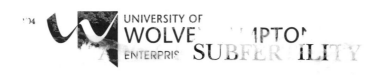

UNIVERSITY OF
WOLVE MPTO
ENTERPRIS SUBFERTILITY

ABC OF SUBFERTILITY

Edited by

PETER BRAUDE

*Professor and head of department of women's health, Guy's, King's, and
St Thomas's School of Medicine, London
Consultant in Guy's, King's, and St Thomas's assisted conception unit, London
Lead clinician for pre-implantation genetic diagnosis (PGD) programme
Member of the Human Fertilisation and Embryology Authority*

and

ALISON TAYLOR

*Consultant gynaecologist and subspecialist in reproductive medicine and lead clinician of
the Guy's and St Thomas's assisted conception unit, London*

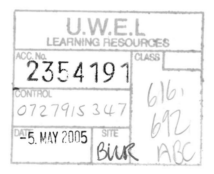
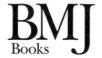

BMJ
Books

First published in 2004 by
BMJ Publishing Group, BMA House, Tavistock Square,
London WC1H 9JR

www.bmjbooks.com

British Library Cataloguing in Publication Data
A catalogue record for this book is available from the British Library

ISBN 0 7279 1534 7

Typeset by BMJ Electronic Production
Printed and bound in Spain by GraphyCems, Navarra
Cover Image shows sperm fertilising egg.
With permission from Alfred Pasieka/Science Photo Library

Contents

Contributors

Alison Bagshawe
Counsellor at the Guy's and St Thomas's assisted conception unit, London

Peter Braude
Professor and head of department of women's health, Guy's, King's, and St Thomas's School of Medicine, London
Consultant in Guy's, King's, and St Thomas's assisted conception unit, London
Lead clinician for pre-implantation genetic diagnosis (PGD) programme
Member of the Human Fertilisation and Embryology Authority

Diana Hamilton-Fairley
Consultant obstetrician and gynaecologist at Guy's and St Thomas's NHS Trust, London

Roger Hart
Senior lecturer in obstetrics and gynaecology, university of Western Australia school of women's and infant's health, King Edward Memorial Hospital, Subiaco, Australia

Anthony Hirsh
Consultant to the andrology clinic at Whipps Cross Hospital, London and honorary senior lecturer at King's, Guy's, and St Thomas's School of Medicine, London

Yacoub Khalaf
Consultant gynaecologist and subspecialist in reproductive medicine at Guy's and St Thomas's NHS Hospital Trust and consultant in the Guy's and St Thomas's assisted conception unit, London

Sadia Muhammed
General practitioner in York, member of the North Yorkshire health authority's expert subfertility group, and former member of the Human Fertilisation and Embryology Authority

Susan Pickering
Senior lecturer in human reproductive biology in the department of women's health, Guy's, King's, and St Thomas's School of Medicine and scientific director of the Guy's and St Thomas's assisted conception unit, London

Paula Rowell
Formerly senior embryologist at Guy's and St Thomas's assisted conception unit, London

Alison Taylor
Consultant gynaecologist and subspecialist in reproductive medicine and lead clinician of the Guy's and St Thomas's assisted conception unit, London

Preface

Hardly a week goes by without some article appearing in the news relating to human fertility. Treatment of subfertility, including assisted conception and its extensions and complications—cryopreservation of eggs, sperm and embryos, multiple pregnancy, hyperstimulation syndrome, preimplantation diagnosis, aneuploidy screening, surrogacy, stem cells, embryo research—bombard the public consciousness through television, the internet, and newspapers. The range of treatments now on offer is bewildering for both patient and non-specialist carer. It is clear from the letters of referral that we receive regularly as part of a major secondary and tertiary level NHS service that there is uncertainty and confusion about what investigations are appropriate, when it is necessary to institute them, and what treatments and advice are reasonable for the general practitioner to offer. Those with infertility are vulnerable to the latest gimmick treatment on offer and may often approach their general practitioners for advice and referral to particular clinics that may be offering what is de rigueur.

With specialist colleagues who are, or at some time have worked or trained at the Guy's and St Thomas's reproductive medicine clinic and assisted conception unit, and with other relevant experts, we have put together a collection of articles that appeared in the British Medical Journal towards the end of 2003. Although largely emanating from one institution, we believe that they reflect modern infertility practice and have special relevance to the legal framework in the United Kingdom. We hope that this collection of articles addressed specifically to general practitioners will be illuminating, and also of use to undergraduates and postgraduates in health care looking for an introduction to this fascinating specialty.

Besides our coauthors without whom this collection would not have appeared at all, we would like to thank Eleanor Lines for commissioning the series and her constant badgering to get the job done, Sally Carter for her fearless and efficient final editing, and Naomi Wilkinson for her efforts to see that the book appeared so rapidly.

Peter Braude
Alison Taylor

1 Extent of the problem

Alison Taylor

One in six couples have an unwanted delay in conception. Roughly half of these couples will conceive either spontaneously or with relatively simple advice or treatment. The other half remain subfertile and need more complex treatment, such as in vitro fertilisation and other assisted conception techniques; about half of these will have primary subfertility.

Most couples presenting with a fertility problem do not have absolute infertility (that is, no chance of conception), but rather relative subfertility with a reduced chance of conception because of one or more factors in either or both partners. Most couples with subfertility will conceive spontaneously or will be amenable to treatment, so that only 4% remain involuntarily childless. As each couple has a substantial chance of conceiving without treatment, relating the potential benefit of treatment to their chances of conceiving naturally is important to give a realistic appraisal of the added benefit offered by treatment options.

Chance of spontaneous conception

Conception is most likely to occur in the first month of trying (about a 30% conception rate). The chance then falls steadily to about 5% by the end of the first year. Cumulative conception rates are around 75% after six months, 90% after a year, and 95% at two years. Subfertility is defined as a failure to conceive after one year of unprotected regular sexual intercourse. It is usually investigated after a year, although for some couples it may be appropriate to start investigations sooner. The likelihood of spontaneous conception is affected by age, previous pregnancy, duration of subfertility, timing of intercourse during the natural cycle, extremes of body mass, and pathology present. A reasonably high spontaneous pregnancy rate still occurs even after the first year of trying.

Age

A strong association exists between subfertility and increasing female age. The reduction in fertility is greatest in women in their late 30s and early 40s. For women aged 35-39 years the chance of conceiving spontaneously is about half that of women aged 19-26 years. The natural cumulative conception rate in the 35-39 age group is around 60% at one year and 85% at two years.

This marked, age related decline in spontaneous conception is also mirrored in the outcome of assisted conception treatment. Recent evidence shows that male fertility also declines with age. Genetic defects in sperm and oocytes that are likely to contribute to impaired gamete function and embryonic development increase with age. The age related decline in female fecundity is caused by a steadily reducing pool of competent oocytes in the ovaries.

Duration of subfertility

The longer a couple has to try to conceive, the smaller the chance of spontaneous conception. If the duration of subfertility is less than three years, a couple is 1.7 times more likely to conceive than couples who have been trying for longer. With unexplained subfertility of more than three years, the chances of conception occurring are about 1-3% each cycle.

Definitions of subfertility

Subfertility is a failure to conceive after one year of unprotected regular sexual intercourse. Subfertility can be primary or secondary
Primary subfertility—a delay for a couple who have had no previous pregnancies
Secondary subfertility—a delay for a couple who have conceived previously, although the pregancy may not have been successful (for example, miscarriage, ectopic pregnancy)

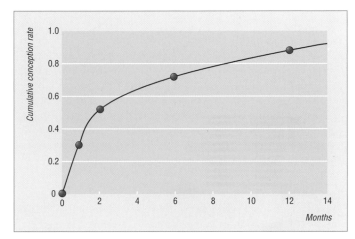

Cumulative conception rate in the first year of trying

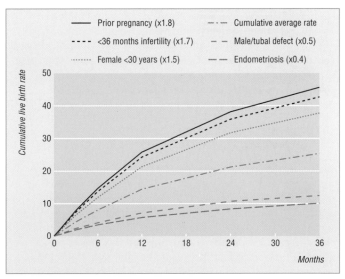

Cumulative live birth rate and prognostic influence of history and findings in couples not conceiving in the first year of trying. The presence of endometriosis, tubal factor, or suboptimal sperm quality may halve the likelihood of spontaneous conception. Data from Collins et al (see Further reading box)

> **Social changes mean that more couples are delaying the start of their family until women are in their late 30s and this brings a substantial reduction in their likelihood of conception**

Previous pregnancy

When a delay in conception has no obvious cause the likelihood of conception is increased 1.8-fold if the couple has secondary rather than primary subfertility.

Timing of intercourse during ovulatory cycle

The chance of conception in an ovulatory cycle is related to the day in the cycle on which intercourse takes place. The window of opportunity lasts six days, ending on the day of ovulation. A study by Dunson et al (2002) showed that the probability of conception rose from six days before ovulation, peaked two days before ovulation, then fell markedly by the day of ovulation. This shows that sperm need to be deposited in the female genital tract before ovulation to maximise chances of conception. This is consistent with the progesterone induced changes in cervical mucus that occur immediately after ovulation and impede the penetration of sperm.

Weight

Pregnancy is less likely if the woman's body mass index (BMI) (weight (kg)/(height (m)^2)) is >30 or <20. Women with a BMI >30 need advice about modifying their diet and doing more exercise to lose weight and they should aim for a BMI <30.

Women with a BMI <20 should be advised to gain weight and reduce exercise if they are exercising excessively. Being considerably underweight is associated with an increased risk of miscarriage and intrauterine growth retardation.

Other factors affecting fertility

The chance of conception may be reduced by smoking, caffeine, and use of recreational drugs. The effect of some of these factors may be attributed in part to an association with other factors that affect fertility, such as an increased risk of sexually transmitted infection.

The effect of alcohol on fertility is not clear as the results of studies are conflicting. Some studies have found impaired fertility in women drinking more than five units of alcohol a week, whereas others have found that low to moderate alcohol consumption may be associated with a higher conception rate than in non-drinkers. Excess alcohol consumption in men can contribute to impotence and difficulties with ejaculation and may impair spermatogenesis.

Is subfertility getting more common?

Fecundity rates may be declining. However, it is difficult to separate changes in social behaviour and trends in delaying starting a family from other factors that might reduce the chance of conception, such as environmental factors. Several studies have reported a steady decline in mean sperm counts over the past few decades in Europe and the United States. They also reported that the incidence of testicular tumours, cryptorchidism, and hypospadias is increasing. Skakkebaek et al (1994) have suggested that a rise in environmental oestrogenic pollutants may be causing these changes.

Major causes of subfertility

The major causes of subfertility can be grouped broadly as ovulation disorders, male factors (which include disorders of spermatogenesis or obstruction), tubal damage, unexplained, and other causes, such as endometriosis and fibroids. The proportion of each type of subfertility varies in different studies and in different populations. Tubal infertility is more common

Factors affecting fertility

Increased chance of conception
- Woman aged under 30 years
- Previous pregnancy
- Less than three years trying to conceive
- Intercourse occurring during six days before ovulation, particularly two days before ovulation
- Woman's body mass index (BMI) 20-30
- Both partners non-smokers
- Caffeine intake less than two cups of coffee daily
- No use of recreational drugs

Reduced chance of conception
- Women aged over 35 years
- No previous pregnancy
- More than three years trying to conceive
- Intercourse incorrectly timed, not occurring within six days before ovulation
- Woman's BMI <20 or >30
- One or both partners smoke
- Caffeine intake more than two cups of coffee daily
- Regular use of recreational drugs

Obesity is also associated with an increased risk of miscarriage and obstetric complications such as hypertension, gestational diabetes, thromboembolism, and complicated delivery

It has been estimated that smokers are 3.4 times more likely to take more than a year to conceive than non-smokers, and in each cycle smokers have two thirds the chance of conceiving compared with non-smokers

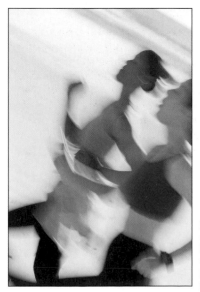

Being underweight and exercising excessively can increase the risk of anovulation, subfertility, and intrauterine growth retardation in pregnancy

in those with secondary subfertility and in populations with a higher prevalence of sexually acquired infections.

The impact of subfertility

The impact of experiencing difficulty conceiving should not be underestimated for couples presenting with the problem. Many find it stressful to seek professional help for such an intimate problem and feel a sense of failure at having to do so. It is not uncommon for the problem to put a strain on the relationship and many couples experience a deterioration in their sexual relationship which exacerbates the problem. General practitioners can provide invaluable support to couples undergoing investigation and treatment and for those faced with intractable infertility.

Preconception advice

If a couple are considering starting a family they may approach their general practitioner for advice on conceiving. Areas for discussion should include things that may improve the chances of conception or increase the chance of a successful outcome to the pregnancy (by minimising the risk of abnormality or of pregnancy related complications for baby and mother).

Managing subfertility

A couple presenting with a delay in conception should be dealt with sympathetically and systematically according to a locally agreed protocol of investigations. Many of these investigations can be started by the couple's general practitioner and completed in secondary care. A cooperative approach allows prompt diagnosis of the problem, after which a realistic discussion can take place about the prognosis—the couple's chance of conceiving spontaneously and of conceiving with different treatment options. Formulating a plan of action with the couple can help ease some of the distress associated with the problem.

The role of general practitioners

General practitioners are often the first contact for couples concerned about their fertility. They can offer advice and support that can alleviate anxiety. Their role includes giving general preconception advice, taking a history, and starting appropriate tests. They should try to see both partners together, although this may be difficult if they are registered with different practices. However, the couple should be encouraged to approach the problem together and must understand that they will both need investigation. General practitioners can also ensure prompt and appropriate referral, and advise on local services available in secondary and tertiary care and local funding policies for investigation and treatment.

Competing interests: None declared.

Preconception advice

Pre-existing medical problems*
- Stabilise medical conditions and ensure that medical control is optimal
- Check that drugs needed are safe for use in pregnancy and do not affect sperm function
- Where appropriate, refer woman to an obstetric physician for advice on implications of the condition in pregnancy

Weight
- Check BMI
- Advise on weight gain or loss where BMI is <20 or >30

Smoking
- Advise both partners to stop smoking

Recreational drugs
- Advise both partners to stop using recreational drugs

Folic acid
- Women who are trying to conceive should take folic acid supplements (0.4 mg) daily to reduce the risk of neural tube defects. Women with a history of neural tube defect or epilepsy should take 5 mg daily

Virology screening
- Screen for rubella immunity and offer immunisation to those not immune
- Consider screening for HIV and hepatitis B and C in groups at risk

Prenatal diagnosis
- Tell older women about options for prenatal diagnosis

Timing of intercourse
- Check couple's understanding of ovulatory cycle and relate most fertile days to the length of woman's cycle
- Advise that intercourse occurs regularly. Two to three times a week should cover the most fertile time

Factors affecting fertility
- Discuss any factors in either partner's history that might warrant early referral for specialist infertility advice

* For example, hypertension, diabetes, epilepsy, thyroid disorder, cardiac problems, and drug history

---

Further reading

- Management of infertility in primary care: The initial investigation and management of the infertile couple. Evidence based clinical guidelines, 1998 www.rcog.org.uk/guidelines.asp?pageID=108&GuidelineID=25
- Balen AH, Jacobs HS *Infertility in practice*. Churchill Livingstone: London, 1997
- Bolumar F, Olsen J, Boldsen J. Smoking reduces fecundity: a European multicenter study on infertility and subfecundity. The European Study Group on Infertility and Subfecundity. *Am J Epidemiol* 1996;143:578-7
- Bolumar F, Olsen J, Rebagliato M, Saez-Lloret I, Bisanti L. Body mass index and delayed conception: a European multicenter study on infertility and subfecundity. *Am J Epidemiol* 2000;151:1072-9
- Collins JA, Burrows EA, Willan AR. The prognosis for live birth among untreated infertile couples. *Fertil Steril* 1995;64:22-8
- Forman R, Gilmour-White S, Forman N. *Drug-induced infertility and sexual dysfunction.* Cambridge: Cambridge University Press, 1996
- Skakkebaek NE, Giwercman A, de Kretser D. Pathogenesis and management of male fertility. *Lancet* 1994;343:1473-9
- Dunson DB, Colombo B, Baird DD. Changes with age in the level and duration of fertility in the menstrual cycle. *Hum Reprod* 2002;17:1399-403

2 Making a diagnosis

Alison Taylor

Couples present at a surgery or clinic because they have not conceived as quickly as they had expected. Some are concerned there may be serious problem that will stop them having a family. Subfertility investigations determine whether a problem exists and enable a rational discussion about options for treatment. The treatment may include waiting for a spontaneous conception. Some of the distress associated with subfertility may be reduced by a prompt and systematic protocol of investigations that allows couples to move quickly to the most appropriate treatment.

Investigations: who and when

Subfertility is defined as failure to conceive after one year of unprotected regular sexual intercourse. Although usually it would be reasonable to start investigations after this time, earlier investigations and referral may be justified where there are important factors in either partner's history.

A woman's age is one of the main factors affecting her chance of conception. The chances of most treatments being successful are reduced substantially after a woman reaches 35 years and become negligible by her mid-40s. Hence, if couples are to gain the maximum benefit from the most appropriate treatment, investigations should be started promptly (after six months of trying if the woman is over 35) and completed according to a locally agreed protocol between general practitioners and hospital providers. Couples can then be counselled about the implications of test results, and a management plan agreed that takes into account the test results and the couple's beliefs and wishes.

At initial presentation both partners should have a history taken and be examined. Regular intercourse two to three times a week should be advised, but basal body temperature charts are not helpful and should be avoided.

A rational approach to investigation

Initial investigations should be completed within three to four months and should establish the following points.
- Does the woman ovulate?
- If not, then why not?
- Is the semen quality normal?
- Is there tubal damage or uterine abnormality?

Both partners must be investigated because an appropriate plan of management cannot be formulated without considering both male and female factors that may occur concurrently. Initial investigations can be started in the community, with the assessment of tubal patency taking place in hospital

Starting investigations in primary care

Does the woman ovulate and if not why not?
The UK Royal College of Obstetricians and Gynaecologists' guidelines include checking a mid-luteal phase progesterone to confirm ovulation in a regular cycle. Time the sample at the correct phase of the cycle (seven days before expected menses). Where cycles are irregular or the woman has oligomenorrhoea (a cycle length of >35 days) or polymenorrhoea (<25 days), ovulation is unlikely and so a progesterone test is of little value.

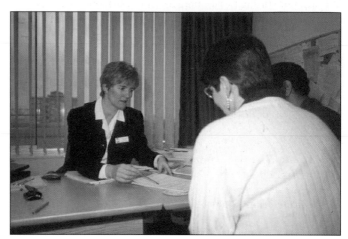

Couple consulting doctor

Factors that may warrant early referral or investigation*

Female
- Age >35 years
- Previous ectopic pregnancy
- Known tubal disease or history of pelvic inflammatory disease or sexually transmitted disease
- Tubal or pelvic surgery
- Amenorrhoea or oligomenorrhoea
- Presence of substantial fibroids

Male
- Testicular maldescent or orchidopexy
- Chemotherapy or radiotherapy
- Previous urogenital surgery
- History of sexually transmitted disease
- Varicocele

*Before a year

> **The female partner of couples presenting with subfertility should have their rubella status checked so that if immunisation is required it will not delay any treatment**

Initial investigations that can be done in primary care

Female
- Luteinising hormone, follicle stimulating hormone (FSH), and estradiol concentrations—should be measured in early follicular phase (days 2 to 6)
- Progesterone test—should be done mid-luteal phase (day 21 or seven days before expected menses)
- Thyroid stimulating hormone, prolactin, testosterone test—should be done if woman's cycle is irregular, shortened, or prolonged or if progesterone indicates anovulation
- Rubella serology test—should be checked even if the woman has been immunised in past
- Cervical smear—should be carried out as normal screening protocol
- Transvaginal ultrasound scan—should be done if there is the possibility of polycystic ovaries or fibroids

Male
- Semen sample for analysis—sample should be taken after two or three days' abstinence and repeated after six weeks if abnormal

Thyroid stimulating hormone, testosterone, and prolactin concentrations need be checked only if cycles are irregular or absent, suggesting anovulation, galactorrhoea, or symptoms of thyroid disorder. Transvaginal ultrasonography is a simple investigation that will detect polycystic ovaries and uterine fibroids. Luteinising hormone, FSH, and estradiol should be checked early in the cycle (days 2 to 6).

Is semen quality normal?

The male partner should have a semen analysis and if some parameters are abnormal, then a second test should be done six weeks later. Ideally the samples should be analysed in the laboratory used by the fertility clinic to which the couple will be referred. More detailed sperm function tests are not needed as a routine part of the initial investigations. The postcoital test is unreliable and is no longer recommended as a routine investigation.

Investigations started in primary care should be completed in a dedicated reproductive medicine or fertility clinic.

Investigations in secondary care

Is there tubal damage or uterine abnormality?

Assessment of a woman's tubal status and uterine cavity can be performed by

- Hysterosalpingography (HSG)
- Hysterosalpingo-contrast sonography (HyCoSy)
- Laparoscopy and dye test with hysteroscopy.

Tests for tubal patency should take place in the first 10 days of a cycle to avoid the possibility, however unlikely, of disrupting an early spontaneous pregnancy. Unless cervical screening for chlamydia has been performed, prophylactic antibiotics such as doxycycline and metronidazole should be given to minimise the risk of infection developing after the procedure.

HSG and HyCoSy

HSG and HyCoSy are "dynamic" outpatient investigations done by inserting a catheter into the cervical canal, after which contrast is injected into the uterine cavity. HSG uses real time x ray imaging to follow the flow of contrast into the tubes and spill into the peritoneal cavity, whereas HyCoSy uses ultrasonography. Both give information about the shape of the uterine cavity. HyCoSy gives extra information because an ultrasound scan of the pelvis is performed at the same time, allowing the detection of fibroids or polycystic ovaries.

Laparoscopy and dye test

A laparoscopy and dye test needs general anaesthesia and carries the hazards of laparoscopy. However, it gives information about the degree of any tubal damage present and enables endometriosis to be detected. Additionally, laparoscopic treatment such as diathermy or laser ablation of endometriosis or salpingolysis or salpingostomy may be done at the same time. HyCoSy and HSG can be used as an initial screen, reserving laparoscopy for patients with a history or symptoms indicating a risk of tubal damage or endometriosis, and for those who have an abnormal HSG. If investigation of the male partner shows substantially impaired semen quality, such that assisted conception treatment (for example, intracytoplasmic sperm injection) is likely, tubal assessment may not be needed. However, information about the uterine cavity may be helpful if ultrasonography shows the presence of submucosal fibroids.

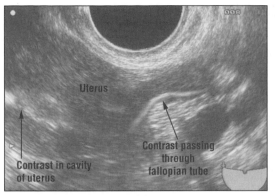

HyCoSy showing patency and flow through one cornu of the uterus

Completing investigations in secondary care

Female

Assess tubal status and uterine cavity

- HSG
- HyCoSy
- Laparoscopy and dye test with hysteroscopy

Male

If azoospermia is present

- FSH, luteinising hormone, and testosterone (with or without prolactin, thyroid stimulating hormone) tests
- Cystic fibrosis screening and karyotype if $<5 \times 10^6$/ml
- Centrifugation of ejaculate and examination of pellet for spermatozoa
- Testicular biopsy or exploration

If oligozoospermia and signs of hypogonadotrophic hypgonadism

- FSH, luteinising hormone, prolactin thyroid stimulating hormone, and testosterone test

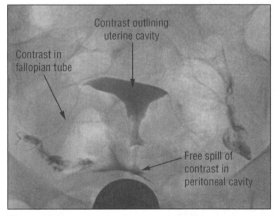

Hysterosalpingogram showing a normal pelvis

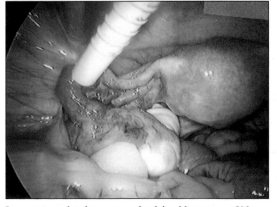

Laparoscopy showing a normal pelvis with passage of blue dye through the fimbrial end of the left tube

Further investigation of azoospermia in secondary care

Where the initial semen analysis reveals azoospermia a centrifuged sample should be examined for sperm in the pellet. Even if only a few sperm can be identified, intracytoplasmic sperm injection can be offered as effective treatment to circumvent the infertility.

If azoospermia is confirmed it is important to distinguish between obstructive and non-obstructive azoospermia.

In obstructive azoospermia, spermatogenesis is normal but there is a block in the epididymis or vas deferens. If congenital absence of vas deferens is suspected, both partners should undergo cystic fibrosis screening because many of these men will carry one of the cystic fibrosis mutations. In non-obstructive azoospermia, spermatogenesis is impaired. This impairment may be caused by testicular failure (so the man's karyotype should be checked and multiple testicular biopsy may show isolated foci of spermatogenesis) or due to a failure to stimulate spermatogenesis by the hypothalamic pituitary axis (hypogonadotrophic hypogonadism). Although rare, this condition should be detected as these patients respond to gonadotrophin treatment.

Interpreting results and discussing treatment options

Female partner

Where the progesterone concentration is low take the following steps.
- Check the length of the cycle in which the sample was taken
- Ensure that sample was taken in the mid-luteal phase—that is, seven days before expected period
- Ensure that other endocrine tests are completed
- An ultrasound scan is valuable to diagnose presence of polycystic ovaries if anovulation is confirmed or the luteinising hormone or testosterone concentrations, or both, are raised
- Advise about weight gain or loss to achieve a body mass index (weight (kg)/(height (m)^2)) of 20-30. This is the key to successful treatment.

A single raised early follicular phase follicle stimulating hormone (FSH) concentration is a poor prognostic indicator for women trying to conceive. It implies a reduced ovarian reserve and the possibility of incipient premature ovarian failure. This is difficult to treat because the response to ovarian stimulation is likely to be poor. Refractory cases may need egg donation.

After an abnormal hysterosalpingogram or HyCoSy, further tubal assessment by laparoscopy will be needed. The main treatment options include:
- Surgery (open or laparoscopic)
- Transcervical tubal cannulation
- In vitro fertilisation.

The choice of procedure will depend on factors such as the degree of tubal damage, the semen quality, and the patient's age. Intrauterine lesions such as submucous fibroids or adhesions need further evaluation by hysteroscopy, at which time they may be resected.

Male partner

Semen samples can vary greatly. If the semen volume is low, check whether collection of the ejaculate was complete. If the first part of the ejaculate, which contains most of the sperm, missed the pot, the results will not be representative.

Investigating azoospermia, by site of abnormality

	Obstructive	Non-obstructive	
	Post-testicular	*Testicular*	*Hypothalamic-pituitary*
Congenital causes	Vasal aplasia, cystic fibrosis, mullerian cysts	Genetic causes, cryptorchidism, anorchia	Kallman's syndrome, isolated FSH deficiency
Acquired causes	Gonorrhoea, chlamydia, tuberculosis, prostatitis, vasectomy	Radiotherapy, chemotherapy, orchitis, trauma, torsion	Craniopharyngioma, pituitary tumour, pituitary ablation, anabolic steroids
Testicular size	Normal	Small, atrophic	Small, prepubertal
FSH	Normal	Raised	Low
Testosterone	Normal	Low	Low

Interpreting results of investigations of female partners

Test	Result	Interpretation
Progesterone	<30 nmol/l	Anovulation: Check cycle length and timing in mid-luteal phase; complete other endocrine tests; scan for polycystic ovaries; advise on weight gain or loss; may need ovulation induction; clomifene should not be started without tubal patency test
FSH	>10 IU/l	Reduced ovarian reserve: May respond poorly to ovulation induction; may need egg donation
Luteinising hormone	>10 IU/l	May be polycystic ovaries: Ultrasonography to confirm
Testosterone	>2.5 nmol/l / >5 nmol/l	May be polycystic ovaries: Ultrasonography to confirm Congenital adrenal hyperplasia: Check 17-OHP and DHEAS
Prolactin	>1000 IU/l	May be pituitary adenoma: Repeat prolactin to confirm raised concentration; exclude hypothyroidism; arrange magnetic resonance image or computed tomogram; if confirmed hyperprolactinaemia start dopamine agonist
Rubella	Non-immune	Offer immunisation and one month contraception
HSG or HyCoSy	Abnormal	May be tubal factor: Arrange laparoscopy and dye test to evaluate further; may be intrauterine abnormality—for example, fibroid or adhesions; evaluate further by hysteroscopy
Laparoscopy and dye	Blocked tubes	Tubal factor confirmed: Possibly suitable for transcervical cannulation, surgery or in vitro fertilisation (also depends on semen quality)
	Endometriosis	Endometriosis: Assess severity; may benefit from diathermy or laser ablation; medical suppression not helpful for fertility May need in vitro fertilisation

DHEAS = dihydroepiandrosterone sulphate;
17-OHP = 17-hydroxyprogesterone

Lubricants for masturbation—for example, soap or KY jelly may be spermicidal and their use should be avoided. If the male partner has difficulty producing a sample by masturbation then a non-spermicidal condom can be used.

Therapeutic drugs that may be associated with impaired spermatogenesis include chemotherapy, sulfasalazine, and cimetidine.

Abnormal semen qualities are an indication for early referral to a fertility clinic, preferably one offering a full range of assisted conception techniques.

Conclusion

Couples who present with subfertility rarely have absolute infertility (that is, no chance of conception spontaneously). Factors that are contributing to the problem usually cause relative subfertility (that is, a reduced chance of conceiving spontaneously) to a greater or lesser degree, and there may be relevant factors in both partners.

Investigations should follow a systematic protocol designed to identify:
- Tubal or uterine abnormalities
- Anovulation
- Impaired spermatogenesis.

Prompt investigation and appropriate referral allow a couple to receive advice and treatment to help them reach their goal of a pregnancy more quickly, and may alleviate some of the distress associated with subfertility. Doctors in primary care can have an invaluable role in starting this process and providing support during further investigation and treatment.

Competing interests: None declared.

Interpreting a semen analysis

Parameter	Normal	Comments if abnormal
Volume	2-5 ml	If low, check if collection was incomplete ("missed the pot")
Count	$>20 \times 10^6$/ml	Repeat sample. Check that no acute illness occurred in two months before sample. Lifestyle advice on smoking, alcohol, and drugs. If $<10 \times 10^6$/ml in vitro fertilisation or intracytoplasmic sperm injection. Refer early
Motility	$>50\%$ progressively motile $>25\%$ rapidly progressive	Repeat sample; refer early
Morphology	$>15\%$ normal shape	Repeat sample; refer early

Further reading

- Royal College of Obstetricians and Gynaecologists evidence based clinical guidelines. *Initial investigation and management of the subfertile couple*. London: RCOG Press, 1998
- Templeton A, Ashok P, Bhattacharya S, Gazvani R, Hamilton M, MacMillan S, et al. *Evidence based fertility treatment* London: RCOG Press, London, 2000
- Balen A, Jacobs H. *Infertility in practice*. 2nd ed. London: Churchill Livingstone, 2003
- Templeton A, Ashok P, Bhattacharya S, Gazuani R, Hamilton M, MacMillan S, et al. *Management of infertility for the MRCOG and beyond*. London: RCOG Press, 2000

3 Anovulation

Diana Hamilton-Fairley, Alison Taylor

Disorders of ovulation account for about 30% of infertility and often present with irregular periods (oligomenorrhoea) or an absence of periods (amenorrhoea). Many of the treatments are simple and effective, so couples may need only limited contact with doctors. This makes it easier for a couple to maintain a private loving relationship than in the stressful, more technological environment of assisted conception. However, not all causes of anovulation are amenable to treatment by ovulation induction. Anovulation can sometimes be treated with medical or surgical induction, but it is the cause of the anovulation that will determine whether ovulation induction is possible. The various options are discussed later in this article.

Causes suitable for ovulation induction

Hypothalamic-pituitary causes

Hypogonadotrophic hypogonadism is characterised by a selective failure of the pituitary gland to produce luteinising hormone and follicle stimulating hormone. The commonest cause is excessive exercise, being underweight, or both. Women who have a low body mass index (weight (kg)/(height (m)^2)) (for example, <20) or who exercise excessively—for example, gymnasts, marathon runners, ballerinas—may develop amenorrhoea because of a physiological reduction in the hypothalamic production of gonadotrophin releasing hormone. Women who are underweight for their height when they get pregnant are more likely to have "small for dates" babies; and children of women who have eating disorders are more likely to be admitted to hospital with failure to thrive.

Sheehan's syndrome (panhypopituitarism), caused by infarction of the anterior pituitary venous complex (usually after massive postpartum haemorrhage or trauma), and Kallman's syndrome (amenorrhoea with anosmia caused by congenital lack of hypothalamic production of gonadotrophin releasing hormone) are rare. Children treated for a craniopharyngioma or some forms of leukaemia may have hypogonadotrophic hypogonadism secondary to cerebral irradiation, which may affect the hypothalamus or the pituitary.

Hyperprolactinaemia is usually caused by a pituitary microadenoma. This leads to a reduction in the production of pituitary luteinising hormone and follicle stimulating hormone. Although the commonest presentation is secondary amenorrhoea, some women may present with galactorrhoea. A smaller number may have headaches or disturbed vision that may indicate a macroadenoma, which needs urgent investigation and treatment. A microadenoma is easily treated with drugs with a subsequent resumption of menses and fertility.

Ovarian causes

Polycystic ovary syndrome is the commonest cause (70%) of anovulatory subfertility. The primary abnormality seems to be an excess of androgen production within the ovary that leads to the recruitment of large numbers of small preovulatory follicles, which fail to respond to normal concentrations of follicle stimulating hormone. Thus, a dominant follicle is rarely produced. Women with polycystic ovary syndrome commonly present in their late teens or early 20s with hirsutism, acne, or

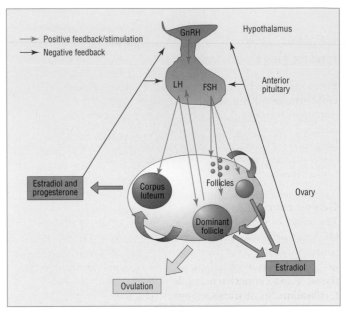

Hypothalmic-pituitary-ovarian axis (FSH=follicle stimulating hormone; GnRH=gonadotrophin releasing hormone; LH=luteinising hormone)

Causes of anovulation suitable for ovulation induction treatment

Hypothalamic
- Low concentration of gonadotrophin realeasing hormone (hypogonadotrophic hypogonadism)
- Weight or exercise related amenorrhoea
- Kallman's syndrome
- Stress
- Idiopathic

Pituitary
- Hyperprolactinaemia
- Pituitary failure (hypogonadotrophic hypogonadism)
- Sheehan's syndrome
- Craniopharyngioma or hypophysectomy
- Cerebral radiotherapy

Ovarian
- Polycystic ovaries

Other endocrine
- Hypothyroidism
- Congenital adrenal hyperplasia

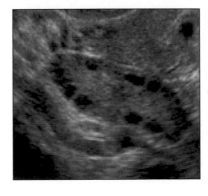

Transvaginal scan of a polycystic ovary. Typically 10 or more follicles of <10 mm in diameter ("string of pearls") are in a single transverse or longitudinal section through the ovary. Stromal density and ovarian volume increase

irregular periods (cycle length > 35 days). Even if they ovulate, the chance of conception for these women is reduced because fewer ovulatory events occur in a given time frame. Only a third of women with polycystic ovary syndrome are obese, but obesity increases the likelihood of a woman with the syndrome developing anovulation.

Causes unsuitable for ovulation induction

Premature ovarian failure (premature menopause)
Unfortunately this is an irreversible condition. The only treatment option that can result in conception is the use of donated eggs with in vitro fertilisation. Patients will need hormone replacement therapy to alleviate menopause symptoms and to reduce loss of bone density (see www.daisynetwork.org.uk).

Genetic abnormalities
The commonest genetic abnormality is Turner's syndrome (45,X), in which underdeveloped (streak) ovaries result in primary ovarian failure (premature menopause). With adequate oestrogen replacement the uterus can grow large enough for the woman to conceive using donated eggs with in vitro fertilisation. Some translocations and deletions of the X chromosome also cause ovarian failure. Information about Turner's syndrome can be found on the Turner Syndrome Support Society's website at www.tss.org.uk

Ten per cent of primary amenorrhoea is caused by androgen insensitivity syndrome (formerly testicular feminisation). These women have a 46,XY karyotype and intra-abdominal gonads that are testes but have developed as phenotypically female because of the absence of, or non-functionality of androgen receptors. The vagina usually ends blindly and, as there is no uterus, pregnancy is impossible. The gonads should be removed because of an increased risk of malignant change. Explaining the nature of the problem to the patient needs care and sensitivity, and longer term psychological support may be needed.

Diagnosis of anovulatory subfertility

Hypogonadotrophic hypogonadism
Regardless of the underlying cause, the concentrations of luteinising hormone, follicle stimulating hormone, and estradiol will be low. A careful history (surgery, radiotherapy, massive haemorrhage, lack of smell, exercise, and eating habits) and a body mass index measurement will reveal the cause.

Hyperprolactinaemia
A serum prolactin concentration of > 1000 IU/l is diagnostic and usually indicates a microadenoma. Magnetic resonance imaging or computed tomography should be arranged to detect whether a macroadenoma is present. Patients with a macroadenoma must have their visual fields checked. The luteinising hormone and follicle stimulating hormone concentrations are usually at the lower end of the normal range with a low estradiol concentration.

Polycystic ovary syndrome
A transvaginal ultrasound scan of the pelvis will confirm the diagnosis. In 80% of women with polycystic ovary syndrome the testosterone concentration will exceed the normal upper limit of 2.4 nmol/l, making this a sensitive and specific endocrine test

---

Causes of anovulation not suitable for ovulation induction treatment

Ovarian failure
- Idiopathic
- Radiotherapy or chemotherapy
- Surgical removal
- Genetic
- Autoimmune

Chromosomal
- Turner's syndrome (45,X)
- Androgen insensitivity syndrome (46,XY)

Investigations for anovulation

Investigation	When done	Interpretation
Progesterone	Mid-luteal phase of cycle (for example, day 21 of 28 day cycle or day 28 of 35 day cycle)	> 30 nmol/l confirms ovulation; if 10-30 nmol/l check when sample taken in relation to cycle length
Follicle stimulating hormone	Early follicular phase	> 10 IU/l indicates reduced ovarian reserve; > 40 IU/l indicates ovarian failure; < 5 IU/l may indicate pituitary or hypothalamic problem
Luteinising hormone	Early follicular phase	> 10 IU/l indicates polycystic ovaries; < 5 IU/l may indicate pituitary or hypothalamic problem
Testosterone	Any time in cycle	> 2.4 nmol/l indicates polycystic ovaries > 5 nmol/l suggests congenital adrenal hyperplasia; check DHEAS and 17-OHP
Prolactin	Any time in cycle (but not after exercise or stress)	> 1000 IU/l indicates pituitary adenoma; needs repeating
Thyroid stimulating hormone	Any time in cycle if woman has symptoms or signs of hypothyroidism or has hyperprolactinaemia	High thyroid stimulating hormone indicates hypothyroidism
Transvaginal ultrasound scan	Oligomenorrhoea or amenorrhoea; raised luteinising hormone or testosterone	Identifies polycystic ovaries
MRI/CT of pituitary	abcboxtIf two prolactin levels > 1000 IU/l	Identifies macroadenomas
Karyotype	Primary amenorrhoea and premature menopause	Identifies karyotypic abnormalities—for example, Turner's syndrome (45,X), translocations, and androgen insensitivity syndrome (46,XY)
Body mass index	Oligomenorrhoea or amenorrhoea	Body mass index > 30 suggests polycystic ovary syndrome; body mass index < 20 suggests hypogonadotrophic hypogonadism

CT = computed tomogram; DHEAS = dihydroepiandrosterone sulphate; MRI = magnetic resonance imaging scan; 17-OHP = 17-hydroxyprogesterone

for this condition. Luteinising hormone concentrations are raised (>10 IU/l) in 45-70% of women with the syndrome.

Management of anovulation

Treating specific causes

Change of weight
Women with polycystic ovary syndrome who are overweight (body mass index >30) should be advised to lose weight. Together with exercise, weight loss (even as little as 5% of body mass) reduces insulin and free testosterone levels, resulting in improved menstrual regularity, ovulation, and pregnancy rates. If a woman is obese when she is pregnant she is more likely to miscarry. Women who are underweight (body mass index <20) should be encouraged to gain weight, and no infertility treatment should be offered until their body mass has returned to the lower limits of normal.

Hyperprolactinaemia
Bromocriptine is safe and commonly used. Treatment should start with a dose of 1.25 mg (taken with food) at night for the first fortnight and then increased to 2.5 mg for another fortnight. The prolactin level should be checked, and if the level is below 1000 IU/l, the dose should be maintained. The side effects of bromocriptine (postural hypotension, nausea, vertigo, headache) can make it unacceptable to the patient. Cabergoline and quinagolide are newer long acting dopamine agonists with fewer side effects. Once prolactin levels have returned to below 1000 IU/l the woman's periods should return and 70-80% of women will ovulate.

Hypothyroidism
In hypothyroidism thyrotropin releasing hormone may stimulate prolactin secretion in addition to thyrotropin releasing hormone from the anterior pituitary. Correction of the hypothyroidism with thyroxine replacement allows thyroid stimulating hormone and prolactin levels to return to normal, releasing the suppression to gonadotrophin secretion and ovulation.

Medical induction

Pulsatile gonadotrophin releasing hormone
Treatment with gonadotrophin releasing hormone that is started in a specialised hospital setting may be suitable for women who have a purely hypothalamic cause for their amenorrhoea, for example women with recovered weight related amenorrhoea but who are still not ovulating. The woman wears a small mechanical syringe pump that can deliver a pulse of gonadotrophin releasing hormone subcutaneously every 90 minutes, and this usually leads to unifollicular ovulation. Local reactions may occur at the injection site. Conception rates are similar to those in the normal population at around 20-30% per cycle and 80-90% after 12 months' use.

Antioestrogen treatment: Clomifene
Clomifene acts by blocking oestrogen receptors in the pituitary leading to an increased production of follicle stimulating hormone, which then stimulates development of one or more dominant follicles. These drugs can be used only in conditions in which the hypothalamic-pituitary axis is functioning—for example, polycystic ovary syndrome. Ovulation induction with clomifene should be undertaken only in circumstances that allow access to ovarian ultrasound monitoring, because of the risk of multiple follicle development and the small but real risk

> **The aim of ovulation induction is regular ovulation of one egg per cycle to avoid multiple pregnancy**

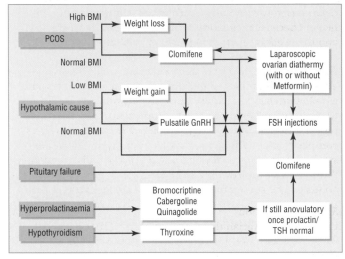

Hormone relationships that may affect fertility (BMI=body mass index; FSH=follicle stimulating hormone; GnRH=gonadotrophin releasing hormone; PCOS=polycystic ovary syndrome; TSH=thyroid stimulating hormone)

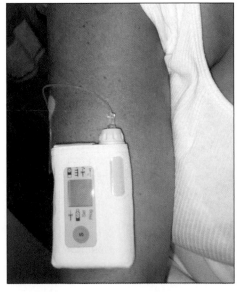

Patient wearing a gonadotrophin releasing hormone pump

> **After publication of a study that showed an increased risk of ovarian cancer in women who used clomifene for longer than 12 months the Committee on Safety of Medicines in the United Kingdom has recommended that women should not take clomifene for longer than six months**

of ovarian hyperstimulation syndrome (Royal College of Obstetricans and Gynaecologists' guidelines, No 3). Seventy per cent of women with polycystic ovary syndrome will ovulate in response to clomifene, with a conception rate of 40-60% at six months. The incidence of twins is around 10%, and triplets 1%.

Metformin

Increasingly, studies report that metformin at doses of 1500 mg a day (in a similar way to weight loss) may improve menstrual regularity by reducing insulin and free testosterone concentrations in both lean and obese women with polycystic ovary syndrome who are not ovulating. However, caution is needed because metformin is not licensed for this indication, and the results of convincing trials are still awaited.

Follicle stimulating hormone injections

Treatment with follicle stimulating hormone is used in women with hypothalamic-pituitary causes of anovulation, and for women with polycystic ovary syndrome who have failed to respond to or conceive using clomifene. As the most serious complications of this therapy are ovarian hyperstimulation syndrome and high order multiple pregnancy, it is essential that this treatment is monitored by reproductive specialists with access to ultrasonography and tertiary care facilities.

Surgical induction

Laparoscopic ovarian diathermy or "drilling" has replaced wedge resection of the ovaries in women with polycystic ovary syndrome. At laparoscopy, five to six diathermy or laser punctures are made in the ovary. Success rates are comparable with follicle stimulating hormone administration, with lower risks of multiple pregnancy or ovarian hyperstimulation syndrome, but complications can arise from surgery and adhesion formation. If too much ovarian tissue is destroyed there is a potential risk of premature ovarian failure in the future, although this risk is still being evaluated.

Competing interests: None declared.

Practice points

- Absence of or inadequate ovulation is a common cause of infertility and in many cases can be treated effectively
- Amenorrhoea and, more commonly, oligomenorrhoea indicate that ovulation is not occurring, so a serum progesterone test is unhelpful
- Weight is important for the success of ovulation induction and outcome of pregnancy. The woman should achieve a body mass index of 20-29 before starting ovulation induction treatment
- Most couples in whom the only cause of subfertility is anovulation can overcome ovulation problems (60-98% cumulative conception rate at six months), but couples with concomitant male factor or tubal subfertility should be treated with appropriate assisted conception techniques
- Ovulation induction should be undertaken in a secondary or tertiary care setting. Couples must be warned of the risk of multiple pregnancy (5-10%) and ovarian hyperstimulation syndrome (< 1%)
- The cumulative conception rate is lower for women with polycystic ovary syndrome than for those who have hypothalamic amenorrhoea

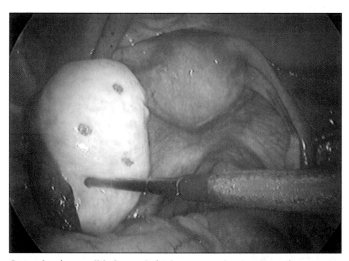

Ovary showing small holes made in the cortex at laparoscopy using a diathermy point to encourage ovulation in a patient with polycystic ovary syndrome

4 Tubal subfertility

Yacoub Khalaf

Patent fallopian tubes are a prerequisite for normal human fertility. However, patency alone is not enough—normal function is crucial. Although patients often view them as either open or "blocked," the fallopian tubes are highly specialised organs. They have a critical role in picking up eggs and transporting eggs, sperm, and the embryo. The fallopian tubes are also needed for sperm capacitation and egg fertilisation. Because the egg is fertilised in the fallopian tubes and the first stages of development of the embryo occur during its four day journey to the uterine cavity, the tubes are also important in nutrition and development. The fallopian tubes are vulnerable to infection and surgical damage, which may impair function by affecting the delicate fimbriae or the highly specialised endosalpinx. A fallopian tube obstruction occurs in 12% to 33% of infertile couples,[1] and so tubal patency should be investigated early.

Causes of tubal damage

Infection

Pelvic infection is a major cause of tubal subfertility. Infective tubal damage can be caused by sexually transmitted diseases, or can occur after miscarriage, termination of pregnancy, puerperal sepsis, or insertion of an intrauterine contraceptive device. The severity of tubal subfertility after pelvic infection depends on the number and severity of episodes.[2] Although a history of symptomatic pelvic inflammatory disease may heighten suspicion of tubal damage, most women with tubal infertility do not report it. Even in women with serological evidence of past chlamydial or gonococcal infections, most are unaware of the infection.

Chlamydia trachomatis

Chlamydia trachomatis accounts for around half the cases of acute pelvic inflammatory disease in developed countries. It is the commonest sexually transmitted agent in the United Kingdom. Chlamydial infections are often not diagnosed because they are usually asymptomatic or have few signs of infection. Both symptomatic and asymptomatic chlamydial infections can damage the reproductive tract. In women, they can cause urethritis, cervicitis, endometritis, and salpingitis, which may result in peritubal adhesions. These adhesions may cause subfertility, ectopic pregnancy, and chronic pelvic pain. Delayed treatment increases the risk of these sequelae and transmission of the infection to sexual partners.

Gonorrhoea

Gonorrhoea is particularly common in young, urban women of low socioeconomic groups and in people who have several sexual partners. It may present as a localised infection of the lower genital tract, as an invasive infection of the upper genital tract, or as disseminated disease with systemic manifestations; however, it may be asymptomatic. Infection with chlamydia is concurrent in 30-50% of patients from whom gonococcus is isolated.

Genital tuberculosis

Genital tuberculosis can cause simple tubal block, tubo-ovarian abscesses, or dense pelvic adhesions (frozen pelvis).

> **Incidence of tubal occlusion rises with the number of pelvic infections the patient has had**

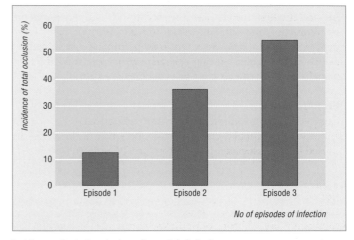

Incidence of tubal occlusion after pelvic infection

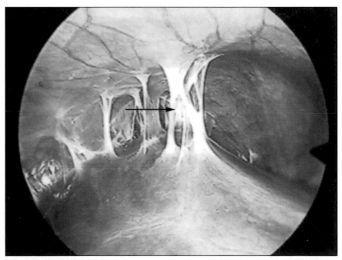

Perihepatic adhesions (arrow) seen at laparoscopy usually associated with pelvic gonorrhoeal or chlamydial infection (Fitz-Hugh-Curtis syndrome)

> **Genital tuberculosis is more common in UK inner city areas with increasing immigrant populations**

Post-pregnancy sepsis

Post-pregnancy sepsis (post-abortion and puerperal infection) may be associated with salpingitis and endometritis. Endometritis with retained products of pregnancy followed by vigorous curettage can result in denudation of the endometrium; intrauterine adhesions (synechiae) can form, which may wholly or partially occlude the uterine cavity. This is an unusual, but important, cause of infertility (Asherman's syndrome), and the patient generally presents with oligomenorrhoea or amenorrhoea, although the hormone profile of the patient is normal.

Intrauterine contraceptive devices

Upper genital tract infection associated with intrauterine contraceptive devices is temporally linked to the insertion of the device. Increased risk occurs in the first 20 days after insertion. Beyond the first month after insertion the risk of upper genital tract infection is small. The risk of infertility after the use of an intrauterine contraceptive device is stopped is not increased, nor is fertility impaired even when the device is removed (usually because of complications, such as menorrhagia).

Endometriosis

Complete tubal occlusion is rarely caused by pelvic endometriosis. Tubal distortion and limitation of fimbrial mobility caused by the associated pelvic adhesions is more likely.

Surgery

Complications after surgery

Previous laparotomy is a recognised risk factor for tubal subfertility, but a history of perforated appendix in childhood does not seem to have a long term negative effect on female fertility.

Sterilisation

People who change their mind after tubal interruption and wish to conceive can have surgical reconstruction of the fallopian tubes or in vitro fertilisation. The results of surgical reversal will depend on the method used to perform the sterilisation (clips, rings, diathermy, or excision), the site of sterilisation, the length of tube remaining, and ovulatory and sperm factor.

Prevention of tubal damage

Practising safe sex is important in reducing sexually transmitted diseases and their sequelae. Screening women of reproductive age for chlamydial infection has been shown to reduce its prevalence and the incidence of pelvic inflammatory disease. Aggressive treatment of suspected pelvic inflammatory disease reduces late sequelae.[3]

The sexual partners of patients must be treated rapidly to decrease the risk of reinfection. The management of women undergoing induced abortion should include a strategy for minimising the risk of post-abortion pelvic inflammatory disease. Women undergoing invasive uterine procedures (hysteroscopy, hysterosalpingo-contrast sonography, and hysterosalpingography) should be screened for chlamydia or receive prophylactic antibiotics.

Diagnosis of tubal subfertility

Infection screening

Chlamydia antibody testing is a simple and cheap screening test for the likelihood of tubal subfertility. The predictive value of testing will depend on the cut-off level of the immunoglobulin G

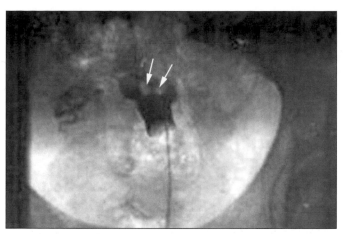

Hysterosalpingogram showing contrast filling defects caused by intrauterine adhesions. The arrows show the areas of front to back adhesion partially occluding the cavity and disrupting the normal endometrium

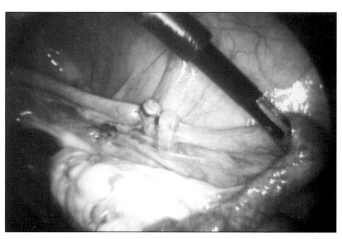

Laparoscopy showing two Filshie clips on the right fallopian tube. Double application has no benefit as it is no more effective and destroys a greater length of tube, making reversal less likely to be successful

The 31st Royal College of Obstetricians and Gynaecologists Study Group on the Prevention of Pelvic Infection recommended that non-pregnant women under 35 years undergoing uterine instrumentation (for example, intrauterine contraceptive device insertion, infertility laparoscopy, hysteroscopy, or endometrial sampling) should be screened for relevant organisms using a sensitive technique before the procedure, or failing that, should receive appropriate prophylactic antibiotics

Suitable antibiotics for prophylaxis after invasive uterine procedures

- Doxycycline 100 mg orally, twice daily for a week
- Ofloxacin 400 mg orally twice daily plus clindamycin 450 mg orally four times daily or metronidazole 500 mg orally twice daily, all for a week

titre chosen and the criteria applied for tubal factor subfertility. Recent studies concluded that the optimum cut-off titre should be 16 because it gives the best combination of sensitivity and specificity. However, high titres of chlamydial antibodies in infertile women indicate the need for early laparoscopy to assess tubal status.

Hysterosalpingo-contrast sonography

Hysterosalpingo-contrast sonography is a simple outpatient procedure using ultrasonography. An echocontrast fluid is introduced into the uterine cavity via a 5 French cervical balloon catheter so that the uterine cavity, ovaries, and fallopian tube patency can be assessed accurately. The use of transvaginal ultrasonography avoids exposure to x rays and is particularly suitable as a diagnostic test in patients with a low likelihood of tubal disease. Finding a normal cavity and bilateral fill and spill of contrast is reassuring, but where there is doubt, hysterosalpingography or a laparoscopy and dye hydrotubation test should be done. Transvaginal ultrasonography can sometimes be useful in detecting hydrosalpinges.

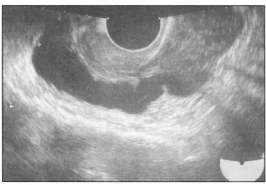

A dilated hydrosalpinx diagnosed by sonohysterography. The sausage shaped, dark hydosalpinx (filled with saline) stands out clearly against background structures

Hysterosalpingography

Hysterosalpingography is a simple, safe, and inexpensive x ray based contrast study of the uterine cavity and the fallopian tubes with a 65% sensitivity and 83% specificity for detecting tubal blockage.

Proximal tubal occlusion can be associated with mild peritoneal endometriosis. The mechanism is unclear, but the occlusion is thought to be caused by a combination of the deposition of intraluminal debris from retrograde menstruation and raised tubal perfusion pressure.[4]

Distal tubal blockage, which is commonly caused by pelvic inflammatory disease, is usually associated with distension of the ampullary portion of the fallopian tube (hydrosalpinges) and variable degree of loss of the internal mucosal folds.

Laparoscopy and dye hydrotubation test

A laparoscopy and dye hydrotubation ("lap and dye") test is the most reliable, albeit expensive, tool used to diagnose tubal subfertility. It is usually performed as a day case surgical procedure under general anaesthesia. When there is no prior information about the uterine cavity, the test can be combined with hysteroscopy for maximum information. Morphological abnormalities of the fallopian tubes can be seen directly, and the general pelvic appearance may give some clue as to the likely cause of any abnormalities found. When comparing hysterosalpingography with laparoscopy, keep in mind that both procedures provide more information than on the condition of the fallopian tubes alone. Hysterosalpingography

> An expert advisory group of the chief medical officer for England supported opportunistic screening for chlamydia in sexually active women under 25 years, and in older women who have a new sexual partner or have had two or more partners in the past year

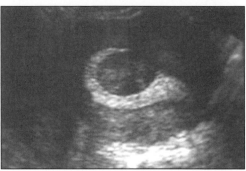

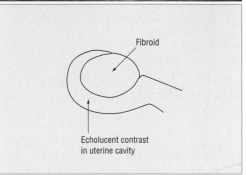

Hysterosonogram showing an intracavity fibroid outlined by ultrasonic contrast medium

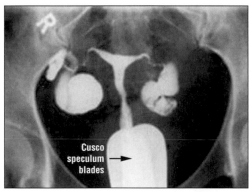

Hysterosalpinogram showing bilateral hydrosalpinges filled with x ray contrast that has been instilled via the cervix. The Cusco speculum blades and the thread of the metal cannula are seen at the base of the picture

Comparison of hysterosalpingography with laparoscopy

Hysterosalpingography	Laparoscopy and dye hydrotubation
• Outpatient procedure	• Day surgery procedure
• Analgesia adequate	• General anaesthesia required
• Simple, inexpensive	• Expensive
• Gives uterine cavity information	• Shows outer contour of the uterus only (unless with hysteroscopy)
• Tubal patency tested	• Shows appearance of tubes and their patency; also appearance of ovaries and pelvic peritoneum
• Screening test	• Definitive test
• Not particularly sensitive for mild distal tubal disease or endometriosis	• Distal tubal disease or endometriosis can be diagnosed and treated

provides information about the status of the uterine cavity, whereas laparoscopy allows inspection of the intra-abdominal cavity, excludes peritoneal disease, and allows laparoscopic surgery. The latter has become especially important because it was recently shown that laparoscopic treatment of early endometriosis improves fertility prospects by 13% over the next nine months.

Management options

"Expectant" management
Patients with tubal subfertility still have a chance (albeit reduced) of natural conception, but this will depend on the extent of the damage. Patients with severe tubal disease can become pregnant while they are on waiting lists for in vitro fertilisation. However, treatment with in vitro fertilisation or tubal surgery is more effective than "expectant" management.

Transcervical tubal cannulation
Transcervical tubal cannulation is an outpatient procedure indicated in cases of proximal occlusion. In 80-90% of cases it is successful in restoring the patency of at least one fallopian tube. About 30% of patients get pregnant in the first three to six months after the procedure.[5] Because of its simplicity, transcervical tubal cannulation should be considered as a first line treatment for patients with proximal occlusion.

Surgery
Surgical treatment and its outcome are related to the site and extent of tubal damage. Reversal of tubal ligation is one of the main indications for tubal microsurgery. Laparoscopic adhesiolysis has the best results if the adhesions are the only factor responsible for subfertility. Distal tubal occlusion may be treated using a laser or more traditional instruments to open the phimosed fimbrial end. Where the tubes are irreversibly damaged and there are large, communicating hydrosalpinges, salpingectomy (laparoscopic or open) is recommended as the success of in vitro fertilisation is impaired by their presence.

In vitro fertilisation
As in vitro fertilisation can achieve a higher chance of pregnancy for all types of tubal subfertility, it should be regarded as effective treatment. Couples should be referred early because in vitro fertilisation success is strongly related to age. However, about 20% of pregnancies resulting from in vitro fertilisation are multiple pregnancies, with attendant risks and complications.

Competing interests: None declared.

1 Hull MG, Glazener CM, Kelly NJ, Conway DI, Foster PA, Hinton RA, et al. Population study of causes, treatment, and outcome of infertility. *BMJ* 1985;291:1693-7.

2 Collins JA, Wrixon W, Janes LB, Wilson EH. Treatment-independent pregnancy among infertile couples. *N Engl J Med* 1983;309:1201-6.

3 Centers for Disease Control and Prevention. Pelvic inflammatory disease: guidelines for prevention and management. *Morb Mortal Wkly Rep* 1991:1-33.

4 Karande VC, Pratt DE, Rao R, Balin M, Gleicher N. Elevated tubal perfusion pressures during selective salpinography are highly suggestive of tubal endometriosis. *Fertil Steril* 1995;64:1070-3.

5 Woolcot R, Petchpud A, O'Donnell P, Stanger J. Differential impact on pregnancy rate of selective salpingography, tubal catheterization and wire-guide recanalization in the treatment of proximal fallopian tube obstruction. *Hum Reprod* 1995;10:1423-6.

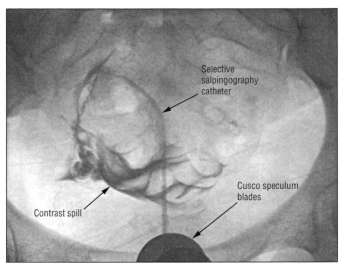

X ray film of a patent fallopian tube after transcervical tubal cannulation. The selective salpingography cannula points at the right cornu and contrast spills through into the pelvis

Main issues in tubal subfertility
- Problems with fallopian tubes are responsible for up to one third of cases of female subfertility
- Major damage to the fallopian tubes can occur after infection or abdominal surgery
- Prophylactic antibiotics given at uterine instrumentation are effective in reducing pelvic inflammatory disease and tubal damage
- Tubal damage cannot be excluded by the lack of a history of pelvic inflammation
- The number and severity of the episodes of pelvic inflammatory disease are strongly correlated with the degree of tubal damage
- Measurement of serum *C trachomatis* antibody titres may be useful in identifying patients with high likelihood of tubal damage
- Hysterosalpingo-contrast sonography is a useful test to confirm tubal patency and to assess uterine cavity and ovarian morphology without exposure to x rays
- Hysterosalpingography is a simple, safe, inexpensive x ray contrast study for assessing the uterine cavity and fallopian tubes
- The laparoscopy and dye hydrotubation test is useful in the diagnosis of peritubal adhesions and endometriosis, and for the accurate assessment of the optimal management options and prognosis
- Hysterosalpingo-contrast sonography, hysterosalpingography, and laparoscopy and dye hydrotubation tests play complementary roles in the investigation of subfertility in women
- In vitro fertilisation is more effective in all cases of tubal damage than tubal surgery, which is only suitable for peritubal adhesions, reversal of sterilisation, and tubocornual anastomosis in selected cases and selected centres with appropriate expertise

5 Male subfertility

Anthony Hirsh

Abnormal semen quality or sexual dysfunction are contributing factors in about half of subfertile couples. As natural pregnancy is substantially reduced in these cases, the man should be assessed by an appropriately trained gynaecologist specialising in reproductive medicine, a urandrologist, or clinical andrologist. Subfertile men often defer consultations because they perceive subfertility as a threat to their masculinity. Consultations should help them to distinguish between fertility and virility, which may ease their anxiety. However, achievement of a wanted pregnancy is more likely to restore manly feelings.

Causes of male subfertility

Subfertility affects one in 20 men. Idiopathic oligoastheno-teratozoospermia is the commonest cause of male subfertility. Although sexual function is normal, there is a reduced count of mainly dysfunctional spermatozoa. Reduced fertilising capacity is related to raised concentrations of reactive oxygen species in semen, which may damage the cell membrane. Abnormal sperm morphology—an indicator of deranged sperm production or maturation—is also associated with reduced fertilising capacity. Less common types of male subfertility are caused by testicular or genital tract infection, disease, or abnormalities. Systemic disease, external factors (such as drugs, lifestyle, etc), or combinations of these also result in male subfertility. Male subfertility is rarely caused by endocrine deficiency.

Falling sperm counts have not affected global fertility, although the theory of increased oestrogenic compounds in drinking water is of concern because the incidence of cryptorchidism and testicular cancer is increasing.

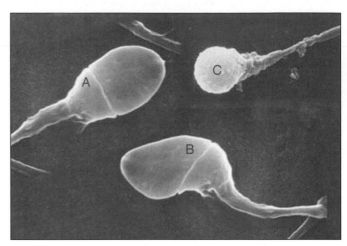

Sperm morphology is related to the fertilising capacity by in vitro fertilisation. (A=normal sperm head; B=abnormal head; C=globozoospermia—a rare syndrome in which all sperm heads lack acrosome caps and cannot fertilise)

Semen analysis is the cornerstone of male fertility assessment and is often the trigger to refer patients for a specialist opinion. Semen samples are best sent to laboratories linked with infertility services. Ideally two samples around six weeks apart (unless the first is unequivocally normal) are required. The samples should be produced by masturbation after three days' abstinence. Men may use non-spermicidal condoms if they have difficulty with, or religious objections to, masturbation

Semen analysis terminology

- Normozoospermia—All semen parameters normal
- Oligozoospermia—Reduced sperm numbers
    Mild to moderate: 5-20 million/ml of semen
    Severe: <5 million/ml of semen
- Asthenozoospermia—Reduced sperm motility
- Teratozoospermia—Increased abnormal forms of sperm
- Oligoasthenoteratozoospermia—Sperm variables all subnormal
- Azoospermia—No sperm in semen
- Aspermia (anejaculation)—No ejaculate (ejaculation failure)
- Leucocytospermia—Increased white cells in semen
- Necrozoospermia—All sperm are non-viable or non-motile

Normal seminal fluid analysis (World Health Organization, 1999)

- Volume >2 ml
- Sperm concentration >20 million/ml
- Sperm motility >50% progressive or >25% rapidly progressive
- Morphology (strict criteria) >15% normal forms
- White blood cells <1 million/ml
- Immunobead or mixed antiglobulin reaction test* <50%

*Tests for the presence of antibodies coating the sperm

Clinical assessment

History taking should include the frequency of coitus, erectile function, ejaculation, scrotal disorders or surgery, urinary symptoms, past illnesses, lifestyle factors, and any drugs taken. Physical examination should seek signs of hypogonadism (small testes), hypoandrogenism (lack of facial and body hair), systemic disease, and abnormalities of the penis or testicles. Testicular sizes are assessed by length (cm) or volume (ml) and are measured with an orchidometer. Because of the risk of cancer, a urological opinion is essential if there is an intratesticular lump or the testes are undescended or absent. Scrotal ultrasonography is helpful in confirming a varicocele or

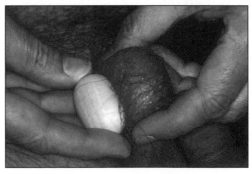

A simple orchidometer is a 4 cm long (20 ml) ovoid used to assess testis size in subfertile men. Normal testes are more than 4 cm and firm in consistency. Abnormal testes are soft and smaller. Both testes should be carefully examined to exclude a tumour

testicular tumour. Transrectal ultrasonography of the prostate may identify the cause of a low volume ejaculate. Serum follicle stimulating hormone is a useful index of impaired spermatogenesis. Genetic screening (karyotype, or DNA analysis for Y chromosome microdeletions or cystic fibrosis) is indicated for men with severe oligozoospermia and most men with azoospermia.

Treatment options for subfertile men

As all couples hope and prefer to conceive naturally, a specific diagnosis should be sought and corrected where appropriate. However, a couple with subfertility of longer than three years, or with a non-reversible form of subfertility is unlikely to conceive spontaneously and should join an assisted conception programme without delay.

What doesn't work

- Abstaining from coitus until ovulation does not improve the semen or likelihood of conception. Increasing coital frequency (alternate days) supplies more viable spermatozoa that normally remain motile in the female tract for two to three days
- Treatment with gonadotrophin injections, androgens (mesterolone) or antioestrogens (clomifene or tamoxifen) is not indicated because although they may improve the sperm count, fertility rates are not improved as the spermatozoa remain dysfunctional

Stopping adverse drugs and drug misuse

Several drugs impair spermatogenesis or sexual function. Most common are sulfasalazine and anabolic steroids when misused by athletes. These effects are reversible, allowing fertility to return to normal in six to 12 months if the drugs are withdrawn. Chemotherapy and radiotherapy damage spermatogenesis, hence sperm banking should be offered to male patients with cancer irrespective of sperm quality.

Timing and lifestyle changes

Most cases of mild to moderate oligozoospermia are idiopathic, but transient oligozoospermia can follow influenza or a major illness and improves within three to six months. The incidence of spontaneous conception each month is 1-2% and justifies conservative or empirical treatment for younger couples. The incidence also explains the powerful placebo effect of some treatments. Advice can be given on lifestyle changes and on the avoidance of fertility impairing drugs.

Treating accessory gland infection

With the increased prevalence of chlamydia, accessory gland infection may cause partial obstruction, focal epididymitis, or subclinical prostatitis. Semen cultures are rarely useful but antibiotic treatment (for example, doxycycline, erythromycin, ciprofloxacin) is often given empirically. Antioxidants (for example, vitamins C and E) absorb reactive oxygen species and are purported to improve sperm motility, although no convincing evidence exists that pregnancy rates are improved.

Assisted conception

Assisted conception gives most infertile men the chance of biological fatherhood, and it is most successful if the woman is under 35 years. The method indicated depends on the quantity and quality of sperm isolated from the semen after "washing" or density gradient techniques. The resulting sperm preparations have improved counts of morphologically normal progressively motile spermatozoa.

Genetics and male infertility

Clinical diagnosis	Genetic tests	Most common defects	Incidence (%)
Congenital bilateral absence of vas deferens (CBAVD)	Cystic fibrosis (CFTR gene)	ΔF508, R117H	66
Non-obstructive azoospermia	Karyotype	47, XXY	15-30
	Y chromosome microdeletions	AZFa, AZFb, AZFc	10-15
Severe (<5M/ml) oligozoospermia	Karyotype	47, XXY	1-2
		Translocation*	0.2-0.4
	Y chromosome microdeletions	Partial AZFb, AZFc	7-10

CFTR = cystic fibrosis transmembrane conductance regulator;
AZF = azoospermia factor: AZFa and AZFb cause severe defects of spermatogenesis; AZFc causes mild defects of spermatogenesis and contains the DAZ (Deleted in AZoospermia) gene family.
47,XXY = Klinefelter's syndrome
*Autosomal Robertsonian or balanced reciprocal translocation

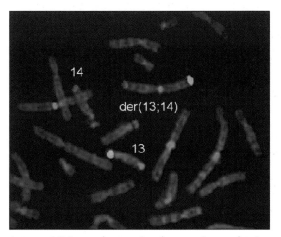
Autosomal Robertsonian translocations may be associated with poor sperm quality and subfertility

Drugs that can impair male fertility

- Impaired spermatogenesis—Sulfasalazine, methotrexate, nitrofurantoin, colchicine, chemotherapy
- Pituitary suppression—Testosterone injections, gonadotrophin releasing hormone analogues
- Antiandrogenic effects—Cimetidine, spironolactone
- Ejaculation failure—α blockers, antidepressants, phenothiazines
- Erectile dysfunction—β blockers, thiazide diuretics, metoclopramide
- Drugs of misuse—Anabolic steroids, cannabis, heroin, cocaine

Conservative measures for men with suboptimal semen analyses

- Stop smoking—Nicotine reduces seminal plasma antioxidants
- Have frequent intercourse—Increases output of non-senile spermatozoa
- Reduce alcohol intake—Alcohol can suppress spermatogenesis
- Wear boxer shorts and avoid hot baths—Heat suppresses spermatogenesis
- Avoid pesticides, herbicides, heat, and radiation at work—All impair spermatogenesis

Intrauterine insemination

In mild or moderate oligozoospermia some spermatozoa are functionally normal. Intrauterine insemination is feasible with preparations of three to five million progressively motile sperm. The woman must have at least one normal patent fallopian tube for successful interuterine insemination. Without ovarian stimulation, three to six cycles of intrauterine insemination result in conception in 15-30% of couples.

In vitro fertilisation and intracytoplasmic sperm injection

A prepared sample containing one to two million progressive sperm is required for adequate oocyte fertilisation with in vitro fertilisation. Not surprisingly, fertilisation is lowest when it is the man who is infertile. However, intracytoplasmic sperm injection needs only one viable sperm for microinjection into each egg. The technique is indicated if the semen preparation yields too few normal motile sperm for in vitro fertilisation, as occurs in severe oligozoospermia. Intracytoplasmic sperm injection is appropriate after unexpectedly, poor, or absent fertilisation in vitro. It is also an effective technique for men with azoospermia by using spermatozoa that have been surgically retrieved from the epididymis or testis.

Severe oligoasthenoteratozoospermia

Most cases of severe oligoasthenoteratozoospermia are caused by idiopathic testicular abnormality or disorder. Genetic tests are abnormal in 7-10% of men with sperm counts less than 5 million/ml. Severely impaired sperm motility may be caused by antibodies, chronic prostatitis, or rare recessive intrinsic defects of the sperm tail linked to sinopulmonary disease (for example, Kartagener's syndrome). Treatment of severe oligoasthenoteratozoospermia rarely improves the semen quality, but intracytoplasmic sperm injection is often successful even if only few weakly motile spermatozoa can be isolated from the ejaculate.

Azoospermia

Azoospermia (absence of sperm from the semen) can be caused by hypothalamic-pituitary failure, testicular failure, or testicular obstruction. Testicular size and the concentration of serum follicle stimulating hormone determine the clinical diagnosis. Although azoospermia is uncommon, 75% of men who have the condition now have the opportunity of biological fatherhood through assisted conception techniques.

Hypogonadotrophic hypogonadism

Hypogonadotrophic hypogonadism is rare but can be treated with gonadotrophin injections or by administering gonadotrophin releasing hormone by infusion pump. Natural conceptions often occur within a year of treatment because any spermatozoa secreted will be functionally normal.

Obstructive azoospermia

Men with obstructive azoospermia have normal spermatogenesis and hence normal size testes, normal concentrations of serum follicle stimulating hormone, and they are normally virilised. If neither vas is palpable, congenital bilateral absence of the vas deferens is diagnosed, which cannot be corrected surgically. As two thirds of men with palpable congenital bilateral absence of the vas deferens carry cystic fibrosis mutations, both partners require screening.

Other cases of obstructive azoospermia occur after vasectomy or they are caused by epididymal obstruction after chlamydia or gonorrhoea. Vasectomy reversal will return sperm to the

> Testing for sperm antibodies is controversial. False positive results occur and antibodies do not necessarily impair sperm function. Antibodies may be found in genital infections and obstructions, but specific treatment is of limited value. Corticosteroids have been used successfully for high titre sperm antibodies. However, severe side effects may occur, including bilateral necrosis of the hip and gastric ulceration. In vitro fertilisation is a more effective and safer way to achieve pregnancy

> Live birth rates of 20-30% per in vitro fertilisation cycle are achievable, even in severe oligozoospermia or azoospermia, if the woman is under 35 years

Varicocele controversy

Varicoceles occur in 15% of men in general and in 30% of subfertile men. Varicoceles probably impair spermatogenesis by increasing the temperature in the scrotum. Achievement of pregnancies is often attributed to varicocele surgery because semen quality may improve after surgery and because conceptions occur in the partners of 15% of infertile men with or without surgery. However, clinical trials are equivocal. Varicoceles can be ligated or embolised, but as it may take one to two years for the couple to achieve a pregnancy, clinicians should recommend assisted conception if the woman is older than 35 years

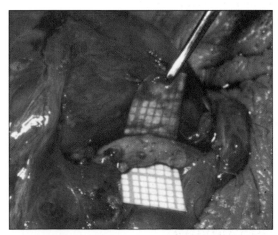

Microsurgical vasovasostomy for vasectomy reversal. Using an operating microscope, the cut and often fibrosed ends of the vas deferens are dissected free from surrounding tissue and anastomosed using fine nylon sutures to re-establish patency. The small squares on the graph paper are 1 mm wide

ejaculate in 80-90% of men, and pregnancies occur in 40-50% of couples in one to two years. Testicular exploration may be indicated for other obstructions because reconstructive surgery results in sperm positive semen in 30-50% of cases, and pregnancies in 20-25% of couples. Sperm retrieved during these reconstructive procedures can be frozen for future intracytoplasmic sperm injection cycles.

Non-obstructive azoospermia

Non-obstructive azoospermia may be caused by cryptorchidism, Klinefelter's syndrome (47,XXY), Y chromosome deletions, chemotherapy or radiotherapy—for example, for lymphoma or testicular cancer. However, many cases of non-obstructive azoospermia are idiopathic. Multiple testicular biopsy may show scattered foci of spermatogenesis in about half the cases with potential for surgical sperm retrieval and intracytoplasmic sperm injection. Men with non-obstructive azoospermia should have genetic testing as 15-30% of them have sex chromosome aneuploidy or Y chromosome deletions.

Surgical sperm retrieval

Surgical sperm retrieval for intracytoplasmic sperm injection is indicated in obstructive azoospermia where spermatogenesis is usually normal, or non-obstructive azoospermia where spermatogenesis is present on biopsy in 30-50% of cases. Results of intracytoplasmic sperm injection using surgically retrieved sperm are similar to cycles where ejaculated sperm is used. Percutaneous epididymal sperm aspiration (PESA) or testicular sperm aspiration (TESA) or testicular sperm extraction (TESE) are usually feasible under local anaesthetic and sedation.

Sexual dysfunction

Most men with erectile or ejaculation failure have normal sperm function and are managed according to whether ejaculation can be stimulated. Men unable to produce the sample for in vitro fertilisation usually respond to sildenafil.

In retrograde ejaculation, where the emission enters the bladder because of non-surgical sphincter failure (for example, in diabetes), oral sympathomimetics (for example, pseudoephedrine) may close the incompetent bladder neck and produce antegrade ejaculation. Retrograde ejaculation caused by anatomical sphincter defects (for example, after prostatectomy or other bladder neck incision) is managed by intrauterine insemination. The sperm that are used are isolated from post-ejaculation urine, which is suitably alkalinised by oral sodium bicarbonate and adjusted for osmolarity.

In men whose spinal cord is injured, semen is usually obtained with a vibrator when vaginal insemination at home may be successful. If this fails, and in cases of aspermia caused by pelvic injury or multiple sclerosis, rectal electrostimulation usually provides semen suitable for assisted conception. If ejaculation is not induced, sperm can be retrieved by vas deferens aspiration for intrauterine insemination or in vitro fertilisation or by testicular aspiration for intracytoplasmic sperm injection.

Donor insemination

Donor insemination is the principal choice for the 1 in 200 infertile men (and their partners) who have no sperm because of traumatic or congenital anorchia or total germ cell aplasia. As donor semen is selected for high quality, the live birth rate of 7-15% per cycle is largely dependent on the fertility of the woman. Adoption is the only other option at present.

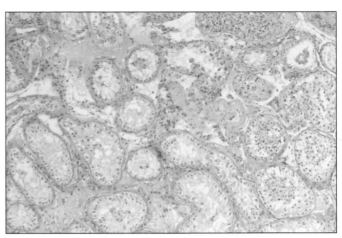

Testicular biopsy of non-obstructive azoospermia showing Sertoli cell only syndrome with a focus of spermatogenesis. All biopsies obtained for testicular sperm extraction in non-obstructive azoospermia are assessed histologically because of the increased prevalence (0.4-1.1%) of carcinoma in situ in subfertile men

Further reading

- Hargreave TB, Mills JA. Investigating and managing infertility in general practice. *BMJ* 1998;316:1438-41
- Hirsh AV. Investigation and therapeutic options for infertile men presenting in assisted conception units. In: Brinsden PR, ed. *In-vitro fertilisation and assisted reproduction.* 2nd ed. London: Parthenon, 1999
- Hull MGR, Glazener CMA, Kelly NJ, Conway DI, Foster PA, Hinton RA, et al. Population study of causes, treatment, and outcome of infertility. *BMJ* 1985;291:1693-7
- Royal College of Obstetricians and Gynaecologists. *Evidence-based guidelines: initial investigation and management of the infertile couple.* London: RCOG, 1998
- Royal College of Obstetricians and Gynaecologists. *Evidence-based guidelines: management of infertility in secondary care.* London: RCOG, 1998
- Royal College of Obstetricians and Gynaecologists. *Evidence-based guidelines: management of infertility in tertiary care.* London: RCOG, 2000
- Rowe PJ, Comhaire FH, Hargreave TB, Mahmoud AMA. *WHO manual for the standard investigation, diagnosis and management of the infertile male.* Cambridge: Cambridge University Press, 2000
- Skakkebaek NE, Giwercman A, de Kretser D. Pathogenesis and management of male infertility. *Lancet* 1994;343:1473-9
- Vale J, Hirsh AV. *Male sexual dysfunction.* Oxford: Blackwell Science, in press

The scanning electron micrographs of sperm morphology are published with permission of Alpha from *Scientists in Reproductive Medicine* newsletters 1996 and 2000. The testicular biopsy showing non-obstructive azoospermia is at a magnification x 400 and is reprinted with permission from Dr K Shah, London.

Competing interests: None declared.

6 Unexplained infertility, endometriosis, and fibroids

Roger Hart

The presence of patent fallopian tubes, normal ovulation, and normal sperm parameters may still be associated with subfertility because of distortion of the uterine cavity or the presence of intraperitoneal endometriosis. Frustratingly, in some cases, no abnormality is found on routine investigation and the infertility is labelled "unexplained."

Unexplained subfertility

A couple is usually referred for investigation of subfertility after trying unsuccessfully to conceive for a year. Although many may despair of ever conceiving, the chance of successful spontaneous conception during the subsequent year is about 50%. However, the chance is reduced if the woman has never been pregnant (primary subfertility) or is aged over 30, or the duration of subfertility is longer than three years.

Diagnosis of unexplained subfertility

Unexplained subfertility is a diagnosis of exclusion. Up to 25% of patients who present for investigation in a reproductive medicine clinic are diagnosed with unexplained fertility. The diagnosis is usually made after investigations show normal semen parameters, ovulatory concentrations of serum progesterone in the mid-luteal phase, tubal patency, and a normal uterine cavity.

A frustrating diagnosis for patients

It is important to emphasise to couples with a diagnosis of unexplained subfertility that they have only had essential, simple fertility tests that do not always assess function. For example, despite showing tubal patency, normal transport of eggs and sperm in tubes has not been evaluated as no test for this is available. Although a woman may have an ovulatory concentration of serum progesterone and this indicates formation of a corpus luteum, it does not necessarily mean that an egg has been released nor that an egg has been picked up in the fallopian tubes. Even for women who ovulate, there is no information about oocyte quality and consequent embryo quality after fertilisation. Despite normal semen parameters, the sperm may fail one of the steps needed to fertilise the oocyte. Some or all of these potential causes of infertility may be avoided by using intrauterine insemination with superovulation, in vitro fertilisation, or intracytoplasmic sperm injection.

Should further tests be done?

Further tests can be done but they seldom alter management. The "postcoital" test should no longer be done routinely as it is unreliable and seldom alters management.[1] What couples want is not so much to find out "what is wrong," but "what can be done for us." Hence, a pragmatic approach to their treatment should be taken.

Treatment options

"Expectant" management

The decision as to when it is appropriate to treat a couple for unexplained subfertility or to wait for spontaneous pregnancy is dictated largely by duration of subfertility, the woman's age, and the couple's wishes. A woman over 35 should be advised to start treatment earlier than a younger woman.

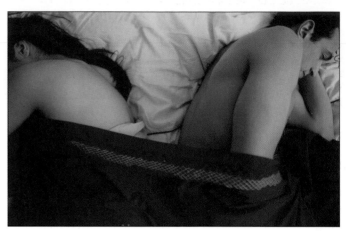

Unexplained subfertility can be a frustrating diagnosis for any couple trying to conceive

> A diagnosis of unexplained fertility can be highly frustrating for patients, who may interpret this as meaning that there is apparently "no cause" for their subfertility and hence no effective treatment

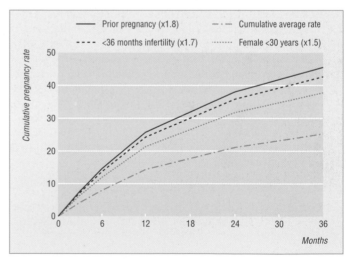

Cumulative live birth rate and prognostic influence of history and findings in couples not conceiving in the first year of trying

> Couples want a baby, not exhaustive and prolonged investigation

Superovulation and intrauterine insemination

Intrauterine insemination with superovulation is favoured as the treatment of choice for unexplained subfertility, although if the woman is over 37 years she may be advised to proceed directly to in vitro fertilisation. Intrauterine insemination is less invasive and cheaper than in vitro fertilisation and can achieve pregnancy rates of about 10-17% each cycle, with 85% of conceptions occurring within the first four cycles.[2] It may be appropriate for couples to have up to six cycles of intrauterine insemination before stopping this treatment and moving on to in vitro fertilisation. The point at which the treatment is stopped will depend on the woman's age, the duration of subfertility, and local funding policies.

Endometriosis

Endometriosis is present in 20-40% of women who complain of subfertility, although it can be found in 5% of fertile women. Mild endometriosis that is not associated with adhesions and tubal defects may be associated with protracted infertility in some women but not others, and it is unclear why. Postulated explanations include intraperitoneal inflammation, immunological factors, unruptured luteinised follicles, and an increase in the rate of miscarriage.

Endometriosis should be suspected when there is dyspareunia, severe dysmenorrhoea, or unexplained abdominal pain, although the symptoms experienced are a poor indicator of the severity of disease. Pelvic examination may show tenderness, nodules of endometriosis on the uterosacral ligaments, or an enlarged ovary, which may be secondary to an ovarian endometrioma. The diagnosis of endometriosis is generally confirmed by laparoscopy. Preoperative ultrasonography is helpful to diagnose the likely cause of a tender and enlarged ovary.

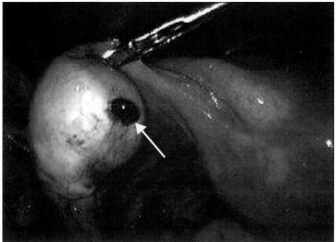

Laparoscopy of an enlarged ovary containing an endometriotic cyst leaking "chocolate" fluid (arrow). These endometriomas develop as endometriotic implants that may bleed slowly into the ovary over months. This patient complained of worsening left sided pain. A small rupture was found and there was a small amount of blood in her abdomen. The cyst was removed and the normal ovarian tissue was saved

Treatment options

Drug treatment to control the symptoms of endometriosis is usually counterproductive to the immediate fertility prospects for a couple. Although some drugs are effective in suppressing deposits of the disease during the course of treatment, most prevent the woman conceiving (for example, gonadotrophin releasing hormone analogues, sequential oral contraception). The woman may even be advised not to attempt to conceive

Superovulation and intrauterine insemination

- This treatment cycle starts with the onset of the menses, with daily, or alternate day ovarian stimulation using injections of follicular stimulating hormone
- Follicular development is monitored using ultrasonography. When one or two follicles are at least 18 mm in size, ovulation is triggered by human chorionic gonadotrophin hormone injection
- The sperm, washed free of seminal fluid in the laboratory, are placed in the uterine cavity via a catheter either immediately or within 24 hours of the human chorionic gonadotrophin hormone injection
- No additional hormonal support is required to sustain the endometrium

Endometriosis is characterised by the presence and growth of endometrial tissue outside the uterus and is often associated with symptoms of dysmenorrhoea, dyspareunia, and subfertility

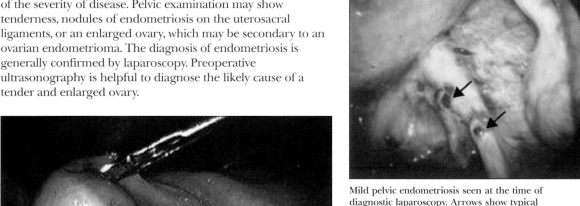

Mild pelvic endometriosis seen at the time of diagnostic laparoscopy. Arrows show typical endometrioic deposits

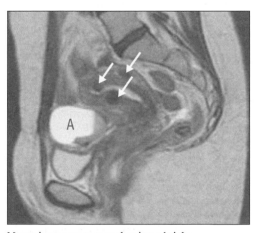

Magnetic resonance scan showing a bright endometrioma (A) with a dependent clot. The arrows show small intramural fibroids

while taking certain drugs (for example, danazol), thereby prolonging the period of subfertility, and with little or no chance of improving fecundity after treatment. Thus, after a period of infertility where endometriosis is present, the choice of approach is surgery or assisted conception.

Where endometriosis is minimal without tubal damage, intrauterine insemination with superovulation may be a reasonable option. For minimal or mild endometriosis, surgical ablation using laparoscopic laser treatment, bipolar coagulation of endometriotic deposits, or excision of the deposits has been shown to be more effective than expectant management.[3] For severe disease the most cost effective management is in vitro fertilisation.

> **Endometriomas should be excised or drained before treatment as (*a*) they may limit the potential of the ovary to generate follicles during the treatment or (*b*) they may inadvertently be inoculated with vaginal bacteria during egg retrieval, leading to a pelvic or ovarian abscess**

Fibroids

Fibroids (leiomyomata) are benign tumours of the myometrium which occur in up to 30% of women. They are more common in African and Afro-Caribbean women, non-smokers, and women who postpone childbearing voluntarily or involuntarily. Most women with fibroids do not know that they are present and have no symptoms from them.

Rarely, women will present because they can feel a lump or a "pelvic fullness" caused by the size of the fibroids. More often they present with menorrhagia or subfertility. Fibroids are more likely to reduce the chance of an embryo implanting if the fibroid is intracavity.

Fibroids are estimated to have a detrimental effect on fertility in up to 10% of cases. They are also associated with an increased risk of miscarriage in women who conceive and half the live birth rate in in vitro fertilisation cycles.[4] Apart from the mass effect, the precise mechanism by which fibroids may cause subfertility is unknown.

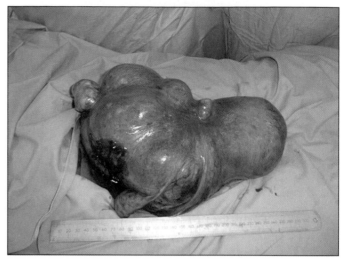

Uterus containing multiple fibroids, which may interfere with fertility even after surgical myomectomy because of distortion of the uterus

Medical management

The size of fibroids can be reduced, albeit temporarily, by administration of superactive gonadotrophin releasing hormone analogues (for example, goserelin, buserelin, nafarelin). The expected reduction in size can be around 30% after four months' use. However, when the fibroids are again exposed to the restored oestrogen-rich environment, they will continue to grow. Consequently a surgical approach is a more realistic alternative. Laparoscopic myomectomy may be suitable for smaller subserosal or intramural fibroids. However, there is still a risk of rupture during a subsequent labour. [5]

Surgical management

If the fibroids are mainly intracavity (submucosal), they can be resected easily hysteroscopically with good long term results for fertility and the treatment of menorrhagia.

However, if the fibroids are intramural, an abdominal procedure (laparotomy or laparoscopic myomectomy) is needed. Gonadotrophin releasing hormone analogues should be used before surgery to shrink the fibroid, to make the surgery less vascular, and often to allow improvement in haemoglobin concentration.

Myolysis—the thermal destruction of fibroids using a laser fibre—is not recommended for women who want to remain fertile. Myolysis carries the risk of adhesion formation and rupture. The success rate of a subsequent spontaneous conception after a hysteroscopic, abdominal, or a laparoscopic myomectomy is about 60% if infertility was the sole reason for the surgery.[6]

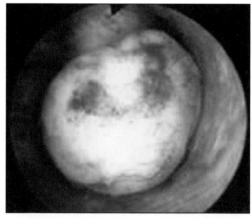

Intracavity fibroid seen by hysteroscopy

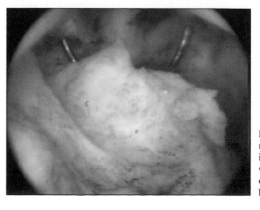

Hysteroscopic resection of an intracavity fibroid, with part of the diathermy cutting loop visible

Fibroid embolisation

Bilateral uterine artery embolisation (fibroid embolisation) is a new technique that has gained some favour in the treatment of fibroids. However, relatively few successful pregnancies have been reported, and there is a risk of hysterectomy because of sepsis of necrotic fibroids. The joint report of the Royal College of Obstetricians and Gynaecologists and the Royal College of Radiologists does not recommend fibroid embolisation for infertile women until more is known about outcome.[7]

Fibroids and in vitro fertilisation

In women about to begin a course of in vitro fertilisation treatment, there is evidence that intramural fibroids reduce the chance of treatment success because they decrease the implantation potential of an embryo. Evidence also exists that the incidence of miscarriage may be increased in women with an intramural fibroid having in vitro fertilisation treatment. However, no randomised trials show whether myomectomy done on these women will increase their chances of conception.

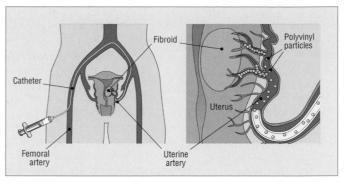

Fibroid embolisation—both uterine arteries are occluded using a transfemoral approach. Small polyvinyl alcohol beads obstruct the blood supply to the fibroids, causing necrosis and shrinkage

1 Royal College of Obstetricians and Gynaecologists. *Evidence based guidelines. The management of the infertile couple.* London: RCOG Press, 1998.
2 Nuojua-Huttunen S, Tomas C, Bloigu R, Tuomivaara L, Martikainen H. Intrauterine insemination treatment in subfertility: an analysis of factors affecting outcome. *Hum Reprod* 1999;14:698-703.
3 Marcoux S, Maheux R, Berube S. Canadian Collaborative Group on Endometriosis. Laparoscopic surgery in infertile women with minimal or mild endometriosis. *N Engl J Med* 1997;337:217-22.
4 Hart R, Khalaf Y, Yeong CT, Seed P, Taylor A, Braude P. A prospective controlled study of the effect of intramural uterine fibroids on the outcome of assisted conception. *Hum Reprod* 2001;16:2411-7.
5 Hart R, Molnar BG, Magos A. Long term follow-up of hysteroscopic myomectomy assessed by survival analysis. *Br J Obstet Gynaecol* 1999;106:700-5.
6 Vercellini P, Maddalena S, De Giotgi O, Aimi G, Crosignani PG. Abdominal myomectomy for infertility: a comprehensive review. *Hum Reprod* 1998;13:873.
7 *Clinical recommendations on the use of uterine artery embolisation in the management of fibroids. Report of a joint working party.* London: RCOG Press, 2000.

The photograph of a couple in bed is from Elinor Carucci/Photonica. The figure showing the cumulative birth rate and prognostic influence of history uses data from Collins JA et al. *Fertil Steril* 1995;64:22-8. The photograph of an endometrioic cyst taken at laparoscopy is reproduced with permission of Dr D A Hill, Florida hospital family practice residency, Orlando, Florida. The magnetic resonance scan showing the bright endometrioma is reproduced with permission of B Cooper, St Paul's Hospital, Vancouver, British Columbia. The figures showing fibroid embolisation are adapted courtesy of Dr J Spies, Georgetown University Medical Center, Maryland.

Competing interests: None declared.

Practice points

- Couples should be referred for assessment of their subfertility if they have failed to conceive after one year of frequent unprotected intercourse
- Unexplained infertility should be treated initially with superovulation and intrauterine insemination except if a couple has more than three years of subfertility or if the woman is aged ≥38 years (in which case early recourse to in vitro fertilisation is recommended)
- Women with endometriosis who fail to conceive should have surgical ablation of their deposits except in severe disease, when in vitro fertilisation is recommended after treatment of endometriomas
- Fibroids are a cause of subfertility. Surgery should always be considered if no other explanation for subfertility is found and is essential if the fibroid is intracavity

---

Further reading

- Buttram VC, Reiter RC. Uterine leiomyomata: etiology, symptomology and management. *Fertil Steril* 1981;30:644-7
- Philips Z, Barraza-Llorens M, Posnett J. Evaluation of the relative cost-effectiveness of treatments for infertility in the UK. *Hum Reprod* 2000;15:95-106
- Templeton A, Cooke I, O'Brien PMS, eds. *Evidence based fertility treatment.* London: RCOG, 1998

7 Assisted conception. I–General principles

Paula Rowell, Peter Braude

Although many assisted conception technologies exist—and have a bewildering array of acronyms—their principal aim is similar. They all aim to bring sperm and the egg close to each other to promote the chances of fertilisation and, ultimately, achieve a pregnancy.

The three main types of assisted conception are intrauterine insemination, in vitro fertilisation, and intracytoplasmic sperm injection.

Intrauterine insemination—Prepared sperm are deposited in the uterus at a time when ovulation is likely or assisted

In vitro fertilisation—Fertilisation is aided by mixing eggs and sperm in the laboratory

Intracytoplasmic sperm injection—A single sperm is injected directly into the egg cytoplasm to achieve fertilisation.

Each of these assisted conception techniques requires three procedures: pharmacological stimulation of the ovary to promote the production of more than one egg (superovulation); laboratory preparation of the semen sample to yield a highly motile, morphologically normal population of sperm for insemination or injection (sperm preparation); and techniques to aid the union of sperm and egg (assisted fertilisation).

Superovulation

Multifollicular development can be achieved by using oral antioestrogens, such as clomifene citrate or tamoxifen. However, more often multifollicular development requires injected preparations containing the pituitary hormone, follicle stimulating hormone (FSH).

FSH used to be obtained from extracts of urine collected from postmenopausal women, which were then purified to various degrees to remove contaminating proteins and luteinising hormone. The extracts provided a preparation of human menopausal gonadotrophins marketed as human menotropins—for example, Merional, Menogon, Menopur. Variation within batches of gonadotrophins, and the increasing unacceptability of injecting biologically derived substances, has led to the more widespread use of recombinant products. These include Gonal-F (follitropin α) and Puregon (follitropin β). Although chemically pure, and thus batch consistent, these are more expensive than the equivalent urinary derived products.

The dose of FSH must be titrated carefully to achieve the desired effect on the ovary without side effects or over-response. Cycles may need to be cancelled before insemination if there is a risk of high order multiple pregnancy. Egg collection should be cancelled if there is a risk of ovarian hyperstimulation syndrome. Better control of cycles may be achieved using gonadotrophin releasing hormone (GnRH) analogues, or antagonists in combination with gonadotrophins. However, GnRH analogues do have side effects such as headaches, hot flushes, vaginal dryness, sweating, mood swings, and depression.

The aim of intrauterine insemination is to provide up to three developing mature follicles. More than three developing follicles would put the patient at risk of a high order multiple pregnancy. For in vitro fertilisation or intracytoplasmic sperm injection the superovulation regimen is more aggressive. These two treatments aim to harvest eggs, fertilise them in vitro then

---

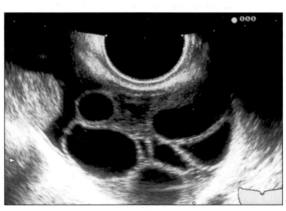

Ultrasound picture of an ovary stimulated for in vitro fertilisation using a more aggressive regimen than used for intrauterine insemination

---

Use of gonadotrophin releasing hormone (GnRH) analogues and antagonists in superovulation

GnRH analogues

- Synthetic GnRH superactive analogues (buserelin, nafarelin) can be administered by nasal spray or by subcutaneous injection. Goserelin is administered by subcutaneous implant
- These competitively, but reversibly, bind to the hypothalamic GnRH receptors. Thus, after a preliminary flare of FSH, all further output of FSH and luteinising hormone is suppressed effectively rendering the woman temporarily amenorrhoeic with menopausal symptoms
- This downregulation of the pituitary gland is used in superovulation regimens to prevent the physiological surge of luteinising hormone and untimely or unwanted release of oocytes, to try and recruit a more synchronous cohort of follicles, and to facilitate scheduling of treatment cycles for the convenience of patient and clinic

GnRH antagonists

- More recently GnRH antagonists (cetrorelix, ganirelix) have been used to prevent premature surge of luteinising hormone during superovulation
- These drugs are administered by injection after follicular development has been started by FSH, and so the menopausal side effects associated with GnRH analogues are avoided

select embryos to be put back in the uterus and freeze any suitable surplus embryos.

The incidence of multiple pregnancy in in vitro fertilisation or intracytoplasmic sperm injection cycles can be controlled by restricting the number of embryos placed in the uterus. In the United Kingdom only two embryos can be transferred, although in certain circumstances three embryos are allowed.

Follicular development under gonadotrophin stimulation is tracked by using vaginal ultrasonography to measure the number and growth of follicles. In some reproductive medicine clinics the rise in serum estradiol concentration is also measured. When the leading follicles have reached around 18 mm, human chorionic gonadotrophin (for example, Pregnyl and Profasi) at a dose of 5000 IU to 10 000 IU is given to mimic the natural surge of luteinising hormone, which induces the final maturation of oocytes.

Sperm preparation

Semen samples are prepared for assisted conception by selecting for a population of highly motile, morphologically normal sperm and removing the seminal plasma, leucocytes, and bacteria.

Freshly ejaculated sperm cannot fertilise an egg until they have undergone further maturation (capacitation). Capacitation occurs naturally in vivo as motile sperm swim out of seminal fluid and through the female genital tract towards the site of fertilisation in the fallopian tubes. Preparation techniques have been developed that select sperm with fertilising ability and promote capacitation in the test tube.

Assisted fertilisation

Intrauterine insemination

For intrauterine insemination, the sample of washed, prepared, motile sperm is deposited in the uterus just before the release of an egg or eggs in a natural or a stimulated cycle. The technique is most effective when it is combined with mild superovulation using gonadotrophins. Intrauterine insemination is usually the first step in treating couples with unexplained infertility. It is simpler, cheaper, and less invasive than in vitro fertilisation or intracytoplasmic sperm injection, and it has few complications. The sperm sample is specially prepared as if neat, unwashed semen was injected it could introduce infection or provoke painful uterine contractions in response to seminal prostaglandins. Intracervical insemination of unprepared semen without superovulation is ineffective as a treatment for unexplained infertility.

When superovulation is used, the size and number of follicles are measured using ultrasonography, and a human chorionic gonadotrophin injection is given to simulate the preovulatory rise in luteinising hormone. The prepared sperm sample is concentrated to a small volume (usually 0.2-0.3 ml) and injected in the uterus using a soft catheter at the same time as the human chorionic gonadotrophin injection is given, or up to 24 hours later. The sperm then swim to the fallopian tubes, where fertilisation may occur naturally if a mature oocyte has been released because of stimulation treatment.

Pregnancy rates vary considerably among clinics but are generally around 15% per cycle. Several factors affect the success of intrauterine insemination including cause of infertility, ages of partners, sperm quality, and duration of infertility. Multiple pregnancy is a substantial risk for superovulated intrauterine insemination, and the cycle should be cancelled if there are more than three developing follicles.

Indications for intrauterine insemination

- Unexplained infertility
- Male infertility—mild oligozoospermia, asthenozoospermia, or teratozoospermia
- Failure to conceive after ovulation induction treatment
- Immunological (antisperm antibodies)
- Ejaculatory failure
- Retrograde ejaculation

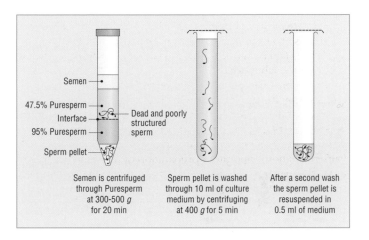

Preparation of sperm for assisted conception: motile sperm can be successfully separated from seminal plasma using density gradients such as Puresperm. Liquefied semen is carefully overlaid on the top of a density gradient and gently centrifuged. Cellular debris, non-motile sperm, and abnormal sperm are trapped at the interface. Motile sperm with normal head morphology move to the bottom of the tube. This pellet is collected and washed twice in fresh culture media. The final pellet is assessed and used in treatment. Samples with low counts can be prepared in this way. By increasing the centrifugal force, sufficient numbers of sperm can be harvested for intracytoplasmic sperm injection

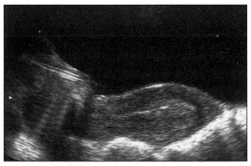

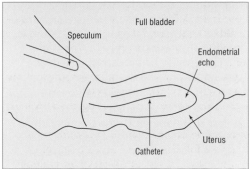

Ultrasound picture of an intrauterine insemination procedure showing plastic catheter inserted into the mid-cavity of the uterus

Donor insemination

In the United Kingdom donor insemination requires a licence from the Human Fertilisation and Embryology Authority (HFEA).

Donors are recruited by sperm banks and are screened for a personal or family history of medical or genetic disorders and sexually transmitted infections including HIV, hepatitis B, and hepatitis C. The donor's blood group and karyotype are tested and a serology test for previous exposure to cytomegalovirus is done. If semen quality is normal, the potential donor should have counselling on the implications before he proceeds. If he does wish to donate, sperm samples are frozen and quarantined pending the results of two further HIV tests three and six months later. If these tests are negative, the sperm can be made available for donor insemination.

For donor insemination, the woman needs to have at least one functioning fallopian tube and she must be ovulatory (or capable of responding to ovulation induction treatment). Insemination is usually done in the same way as intrauterine insemination, by using prepared sperm introduced through the cervix into the uterine cavity just before ovulation. It can be done in natural cycles or in stimulation cycles in which ovulation is induced by clomifene or gonadotrophins. The average live birth rate per cycle is about 10%, but it is influenced by the age of the woman. Most reproductive medicine units strongly recommend counselling for couples seeking donor insemination. Counselling ensures that both partners have the chance to explore all the issues related to the use of donor gametes. Under the regulations of the HFEA only 10 pregnancies can result from one donor.

Gamete intrafallopian transfer

Gamete intrafallopian transfer is a laparoscopic technique in which eggs and sperm are placed directly in the ampullary portion of the fallopian tube, allowing in vivo fertilisation to occur at the natural site. Gamete intrafallopian transfer can be used only in women who have at least one patent fallopian tube.

In common with in vitro fertilisation, a gamete intrafallopian transfer cycle begins with superovulation to recruit multiple follicles and is followed by egg retrieval. Egg retrieval may be done transvaginally (with guidance from ultrasonography). Alternatively, the gametes can be replaced in the tube using a laparoscopic procedure in which the patient is under general anaesthesia. The fallopian tube is cannulated with a catheter containing no more than 60 µl of fluid, which has eggs and sperm in it. The semen sample is prepared before surgery, and a small sperm aliquot containing 100 000-200 000 motile sperm is used.

In centres licensed by the HFEA only three oocytes may be transferred to the fallopian tube with the sperm sample, but two oocytes are more appropriate in young patients. Gamete intrafallopian transfer is not a licensed treatment under the Human Fertilisation and Embryology Act and therefore is not under the control of the HFEA. When gamete intrafallopian transfer is offered in units that are not licensed by the HFEA, there is no regulation of the number of oocytes replaced.

With the simplification of in vitro fertilisation and an increase in its success, gamete intrafallopian transfer offers little clinical advantage. Indeed, the need for general anaesthesia and laparoscopy is a distinct disadvantage. Gamete intrafallopian transfer is used rarely in the United Kingdom now, but more often in countries where there are no or few restrictions on the number of oocytes that can be transferred, or where in vitro fertilisation is less successful.

Competing interests: None declared.

Indications for donor insemination
- Azoospermia
- Severe oligozoospermia
- Failed intracytoplasmic sperm injection
- Risk of transmitting genetic disorder via the man
- Woman seeking pregnancy without male partner
- Couples who prefer a simpler and less invasive approach to treatment than intracytoplasmic sperm injection

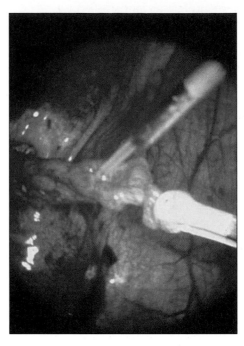

Distal end of fallopian tube with gamete intrafallopian transfer tube catheter being inserted to deposit the eggs and sperm

First proposed in 1984, gamete intrafallopian transfer may be seen by patients as more "natural" than in vitro fertilisation, even though it requires laparoscopy and has an increased risk of multiple pregnancy. Gamete intrafallopian transfer is also deemed more acceptable in some religious circles because fertilisation occurs within the body rather than in a laboratory and surplus embryos need not be created

Indications for gamete intrafallopian transfer
- Idiopathic infertility
- Failed intrauterine insemination, artificial insemination, or donor insemination
- Endometriosis
- Mild male infertility
- Religious objection to in vitro fertilisation

8 Assisted conception. II—In vitro fertilisation and intracytoplasmic sperm injection

Peter Braude, Paula Rowell

In vitro fertilisation (IVF) and intracytoplasmic sperm injection (ICSI) are two of the main types of assisted conception that take place in the laboratory. This article covers these two techniques in detail and looks at their safety and success.

In vitro fertilisation

In IVF, oocytes (obtained surgically from ovarian follicles in superovulated cycles) and prepared sperm are brought together in a dish in the laboratory. Fertilisation takes place outside the body (in vitro = in glass). Cleavage stage embryos derived from these fertilised oocytes are placed in the uterus (embryo transfer) for pregnancy to occur.

The process

Superovulation

Patients receive superovulation treatment with gonadotrophins, usually preceded by pituitary suppression with gonadotrophin releasing hormone analogues (see last week's article). A careful balance is needed to maximise safely the number of oocytes retrieved. Ideally, there should be a choice of embryos for transfer, and some embryos should be available for cryopreservation. However, the risk of ovarian hyperstimulation syndrome also needs to be minimised. Ultrasonography of the ovaries and in some cases monitoring the rise in plasma estradiol concentration are used to check the effect of superovulation. Administration of human chorionic gonadotrophin is scheduled when the leading follicles are ≥18 mm in diameter, and given 34-38 hours before planned egg retrieval. About 10% of cycles are cancelled before the planned egg collection because the response to superovulation is excessive and the risk of ovarian hyperstimulation syndrome is substantial, or, more usually, because the response to ovarian stimulation is poor.

Egg collection

In the past, eggs were collected laparoscopically under general anaesthesia, but now transvaginal follicle aspiration guided by ultrasonography is the method of choice. It can be performed under intravenous sedation and allows access to ovaries that previously were not visible laparoscopically because of severe pelvic disease and adhesions. Most women are able to leave the clinic a few hours after transvaginal egg collection, and the procedure has minimal analgesic requirements.

Each follicle is aspirated in turn, usually through a single vaginal needle puncture for each ovary. The follicular fluid collected from each follicle is examined immediately under a microscope for the presence of a cumulus mass that may contain an oocyte. Once the oocytes have been collected, they are immediately placed in a culture medium containing the essential nutrients and electrolytes required for fertilisation and maintenance of embryo growth. The culture is then kept at 37°C in an incubator usually gassed with 5% carbon dioxide to maintain the appropriate pH.

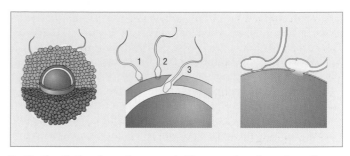

Fertilisation: (left) each egg is surrounded by a complex of cumulus cells (purple) that the sperm need to disperse to reach the zona pellucida, the protective outer coating of the egg; (middle) capacitated sperm first bind to the zona pellucida (1) and release enzymes from the acrosome (2), which digest a pathway through the zona pellucida (3); (right) the sperm is able to fuse with the plasma membrane of the egg and becomes incorporated within the egg

Indications for IVF
- Severe tubal damage
- Bilateral salpingectomy
- Endometriosis
- Mild male infertility
- Idiopathic infertility
- Immunologic infertility

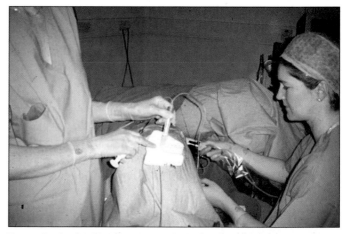

Egg retrieval guided by ultrasonography. Patient is under sedation. A tube carrying follicular fluid from the pierced follicle to the collecting vessel can be seen

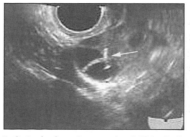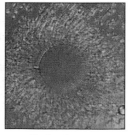

Left: Aspiration of an ovarian follicle during egg collection for IVF (arrow shows needle track). Right: mature oocyte retrieved from a follicle

Insemination

Various systems are used for successful IVF and culture including test tubes, Petri dishes, multiwell dishes, and central well organ culture dishes.

Each oocyte is inseminated with 50 000-100 000 motile, morphologically normal sperm. Fertilisation can be detected 12-20 hours after insemination by the presence of two pronuclei formed in the cytoplasm of the egg around the maternal and paternal chromatids, and by the presence of two polar bodies in the perivitelline space. Fertilisation rates of over 60% per egg collected should be expected, although complete failure of fertilisation can occur because of previously undetected sperm or oocyte abnormalities.

Around 24 hours after insemination, the pronuclear membranes dissolve, allowing combination of the maternal and paternal chromatids (syngamy), which is followed by the first cleavage division to a two-cell embryo. Further cleavages occur at around 24 hour intervals.

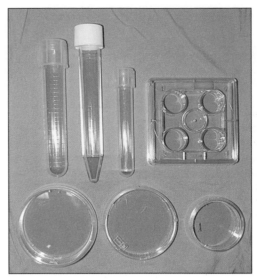

Tubes and dishes used in IVF

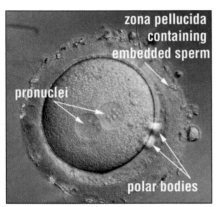

Embryo with two pronuclei on day 1 after IVF

Embryo transfer

Generally, embryos are transferred to the uterus on the second or third day after insemination, by which time they have usually divided into four cells or into six to eight cells respectively. The further on in cleavage that transfer occurs, the more opportunity there is for selection of those embryos that have competence to continue with cleavage both in vitro and in vivo. Although allowing embryos to develop to the blastocyst stage (day 5) may confer this advantage, there are still unsettled concerns about the safety of long term in vitro culture.

Usually two, or occasionally three embryos are transferred together in a tiny drop (< 20 µl) of culture fluid using a variety of soft plastic embryo transfer catheters. Transabdominal ultrasonography can facilitiate the transfer procedure because the full bladder needed for an ultrasound scan tends to reduce anteversion of the uterus. It is also reassuring to patient and clinician to see the fluid containing the embryos placed correctly in the endometrial cavity. The procedure should be painless and the patient may be discharged shortly after transfer. Embryos of good morphological grade in excess of those transferred may be cryopreserved for future use.

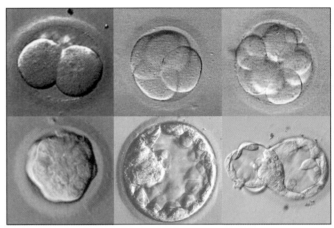

The top photographs from left to right show human embryos in vitro at the 2-cell stage (day 1); 4-cell stage (day 2); and 8-cell stage (day 3). The bottom row shows a compacted morula (day 4); a blastocyst (day 5); and a hatching blastocyst (day 6)

Luteal support

Although in natural cycles the ovary produces progesterone after ovulation, there is evidence of premature luteolysis in some superovulatory regimens. Most IVF centres administer progesterone supplementation via vaginal pessaries, suppositories, intramuscular injections, or oral micronised progesterone tablets until menses occur or the woman has a positive pregnancy test. Alternatively, human chorionic gonadotrophin may be given two to three times a week, but it can promote ovarian hyperstimulation syndome in susceptible or heavily stimulated patients.

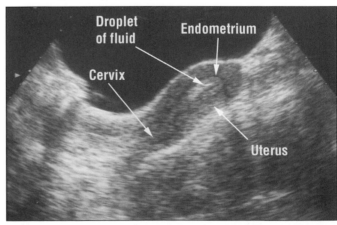

Ultrasound picture of uterus during embryo transfer. The bright spot (arrow) is the small drops of fluid in which embryos were placed

Intracytoplasmic sperm injection

As semen quality reduces, the proportion of oocytes fertilised by in vitro insemination decreases. In cases of multiple defects of sperm (concentration, motility, and morphology), IVF rates may be severely compromised, increasing the risk of the fertilisation failing. ICSI is a highly specialised variant of IVF treatment, in which fertilisation is achieved by the injection of a single sperm directly into the cytoplasm of the egg.

Only mature eggs (those that have extruded the first polar body and hence are at the second metaphase of meiosis) are suitable for injection with prepared sperm. As ICSI is usually used when sperm quality is extremely poor, each sperm can be examined and selected for normality of its morphology before being picked up individually with a fine glass needle and inserted directly into the cytoplasm of the egg. Sperm do not have to be motile but should show evidence of viability. Sperm suitable for ICSI may be obtained from the ejaculate even when few are present. In azoospermic men sperm can be retrieved surgically from the epididymis (percutaneous epididymal sperm aspiration) or from the testis itself (testicular sperm aspiration or extraction).

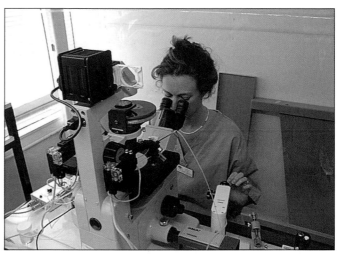

Micromanipulation equipment required to undertake ICSI procedures. The embryologist guides the needle into the egg using joystick directed servomotors

---

Indications for ICSI

Ejaculated sperm
- Oligozoospermia ($< 20 \times 10^6$/ml)
- Asthenozoospermia ($< 30\%$ progressive motility)
- Teratozoospermia ($< 15\%$ normal forms—according to strict Kruger criteria)
- Antisperm antibodies
- Fertilisation failure after conventional IVF
- Ejaculatory disorders
- Preimplantation diagnosis using polymerase chain reaction analysis

Epididymal sperm or testicular sperm
- Congenital bilateral absence of vas deferens
- Obstruction of both ejaculatory ducts
- Azoospermia
- Failed vasovasostomy
- Failed epididymovasostomy

Success of IVF and ICSI

Pregnancy outcome or success rates of IVF may be presented per cycle started, per egg collection procedure, or per embryo transfer. A pregnancy may be defined in various ways: a biochemical pregnancy (a transient rise in β human chorionic gonadotrophin concentration), a clinical pregnancy (a gestational sac and fetal heart beat present), or a live birth. The live birth rate per cycle started is sometimes called the "take home baby" rate, and it is the statistic that all clinics are obliged to make available to their patients by the Human Fertilisation and Embryology Authority (HFEA). All clinical pregnancies and their outcomes have to be reported to the HFEA. The major determinant of success in IVF is the age of the woman. A decreasing ovarian reserve and hence the number and quality of oocytes retrieved continues to decline from age 35 and especially as the woman passes 40. Success rates should be viewed according to defined age groups.

In the United Kingdom, the HFEA publishes an annual guide to IVF clinics, in which success rates are presented according to type of treatment, the overall rate, and the rate when the woman is under 38 years. Success rates in terms of live birth per cycle started, per retrieval, and per embryo transfer are also given.

Before ICSI, the cumulus cells surrounding each oocyte are removed, allowing the assessment of egg maturity. The removal of the cumulus and corona complexes also allows the precise injection of the oocytes, which is required for successful fertilisation. Fertilisation rates are usually 60-70% per injected oocyte when ejaculated sperm are used, but rates may be lower when epididymal or testicular sperm are used

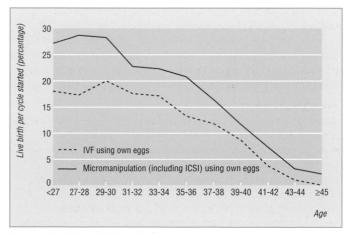

Success with IVF and ICSI declines with age. Data from HFEA's guide to IVF clinics, 2000

Safety of IVF and ICSI

An important aspect of the introduction of ICSI into clinical practice is the concern of genetic and congenital abnormalities in children born after the transfer of ICSI embryos. This is particularly true when epididymal, testicular, or sperm from men whose infertility may have some form of genetic basis, has been used. Available data show that there is a small but definite increased risk to children born of chromosomal abnormality (1.6%), especially if that abnormality involves sex chromosomes. As some of these abnormalities may be inherited from the parents (and the likelihood increases with decreasing sperm quality), it is advisable that men with sperm counts below 5 million/ml (severe oligozoospermia and azoospermia) are karyotyped before they have ICSI. Of more concern and debate is the malformation rate. It seems that the use of IVF or ICSI may increase the risk of a congenital malformation by 1-2%. It is unclear how much of this increased malformation rate is associated with the substantial multiple pregnancy rate and, hence, prematurity rate. However, it seems that even if this is taken into account, IVF babies are 2.6 times more likely to be underweight than those naturally conceived. Further work and monitoring are needed, but the unease emphasises the need for these techniques to be used with caution and only with appropriate indications.

> **The HFEA's guide to IVF clinics is available at www.hfea.gov.uk**

Further reading
- Templeton A, Ashok P, Bhattacharya S, Gazvani R, Hamilton M, Macmillan S, et al. *Management of infertility for the MRCOG and beyond.* London: RCOG Press, 2000
- Winston R, Hardy K. Are we ignoring potential dangers of in vitro fertilization and related treatments? *Nat Cell Biol* 2002:4;14-8
- Ombelet W, Menkveld R, Kruger TF, Steeno O. Sperm morphology assessment: historical review in relation to fertility. *Hum Reprod Update* 1995;1:543-57
- Rowe PJ, Comhaire FH, Hargreave TB, Mellows HJ. *WHO manual for the standardised investigation and diagnosis of the infertile couple.* Cambridge: Cambridge University Press, 1999

The figure showing fertilisation is adapted from Primaton P, Myles DG. *Science* 2002:296:5576. The photographs of human embryos in vitro are courtesy of Dr S Pickering, Guy's Hospital, London.

Competing interests: None declared.

9 Assisted conception. III—Problems with assisted conception

Peter Braude, Paula Rowell

Problems associated with assisted conception can be clinical, ethical, or psychological. This article covers medical problems (such as ovarian hyperstimulation syndrome (OHSS) and ectopic pregnancy), ethical questions that arise from situations such as the creation of surplus embryos, and difficult decisions that have to be made, such as when to advise a couple to stop treatment.

Ovarian hyperstimulation syndrome

OHSS is arguably the most serious risk of treatment with gonadotrophins. It is not clear why OHSS occurs, although it is particularly severe with the use of gonadotrophin releasing hormone analogues and polycystic ovary syndrome. It generally develops if the patient has had an excessive response to gonadotrophins and has produced a large number (20 or more) follicles with its associated excessive rise in oestrogen production. OHSS occurs after exogenous human chorionic gonadotrophin has been administered, or when human chorionic gonadotrophin rises endogenously after a treatment cycle has been successful and an embryo has implanted.

OHSS presents with substantial enlargement of the ovaries, which are filled with enlarging follicles (despite drainage at the time of egg collection) causing abdominal pain, distension, and extravascular fluid extravasation, which results in ascites and haemoconcentration. In the severest OHSS pleural effusions may develop and arterial or venous thromboses can occur because of hypercoagulability.

Superovulation regimens should be designed and monitored to minimise OHSS. However, because of its idiosyncratic nature, the syndrome cannot be avoided completely. Indeed, it can occur simply by using clomifene to induce ovulation in sensitive patients, such as those with polycystic ovary syndrome. OHSS should be managed in a specialist hospital, preferably one with an in vitro fertilisation unit, where there will be the appropriate expertise to deal with the condition. Treatment should be immediate and tailored to the degree of severity. In mild OHSS, without substantial pain or haemoconcentration, close monitoring and analgesia with advice to increase oral fluid intake should be sufficient management. Patients with moderate to severe OHSS should be admitted for anticoagulant prophylaxis and intravenous

Presentation of OHSS

Symptoms
- Abdominal pain caused by enlarged ovaries and acute ascites
- Abdominal distension secondary to enlarged ovaries and ascites
- Feeling unwell, nauseated, vomiting
- Bowel disturbance—can be constipation or diarrhoea
- Dark, concentrated urine because of reduced renal perfusion and low urine output
- Shortness of breath caused by splinting of diaphragm with marked ascites or pleural effusions
- Leg and vulval oedema

Timing
- Early onset: within one to five days of human chorionic gonadotrophin injection, soon after egg collection and embryo transfer
- Late onset: 7-14 days after embryo transfer when endogenous human chorionic gonadotrophin concentration rises after successful implantation

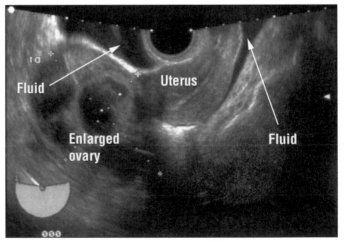

Ultrasound scan showing an enlarged ovary (10 cm x 6 cm) and fluid in the pouch of Douglas and the uterovesical pouch

Management of OHSS

Mild
- No need to admit
- Increase oral fluid intake
- Follow up at regular intervals and report if symptoms worsen

Moderate
- Admit to hospital and assess daily
- Start thromboprophylaxis and maintain until patient is discharged
- Monitor liver function, urea and electrolytes, full blood count, and clotting

Severe
- Strict fluid balance with input of 3 L or more. May need intravenous albumin
- Drain ascites or pleural effusion if symptomatic

Grades of OHSS

Mild
- Symptoms of abdominal discomfort and nausea
- Ovarian enlargement between 5 cm and 12 cm

Moderate
- Manifestations of the mild form, plus vomiting or diarrhoea, or both
- Ultrasonography shows ascites

Severe
- Manifestations of the moderate form, plus clinical evidence of ascites and hydrothorax
- Haemoconcentration, coagulation abnormalities, impaired renal function, hepatic dysfunction, and thromboembolism

rehydration; if they also have a reduced urinary output or have marked distension or breathing difficulties they may require paracentesis or pleural fluid drainage.

Ectopic pregnancy

Patients who need in vitro fertilisation are often surprised that ectopic pregnancy is still a risk even after the embryo has been transferred to the uterus. Among the patients who become pregnant after assisted conception, around 4% of the pregnancies will be ectopic. The embryos migrate to the ostial ends of the tubes after transfer, or they may inadvertently be placed there when they are transferred. The risk of inadvertent tubal transfer can be reduced by conducting the embryo transfer procedure under ultrasound guidance. Patients with prior tubal damage are at most risk, although the possibility of ectopic pregnancy cannot be eliminated in any patient.

Heterotopic pregnancy (a multiple pregnancy with one embryo in the uterus and one embryo in the tube) is extremely rare naturally (1:30 000), but the rate may be as high as 1% in women who have had assisted conception. Thus, this diagnosis must be considered where symptoms of ectopic pregnancy occur, even if ultrasonography shows a pregnancy sac in the uterus. Generally, ectopic pregnancy is detected early after assisted conception because the pregnancy is carefully monitored using ultrasonography.

Multiple pregnancy

Although viewed as a blessing by some longstanding subfertile couples who now have "two for the price of one," multiple pregnancy, especially higher order multiples (three or more), has a substantial morbidity and mortality and is an enormous cost to the health service. Besides the increase in neonatal mortality because of prematurity, the incidence of cerebral palsy in twins is five times that in singletons, and in triplet pregnancies it is 19 times more frequent. The rate of triplet and other higher order births has risen since the advent of assisted reproductive techniques, such as ovulation induction, in vitro fertilisation, and intracytoplasmic sperm injection. It has been estimated that if the triplet pregnancies resulting from fertility treatment could be prevented in the United Kingdom, the money saved on neonatal care could fund one cycle of in vitro fertilisation treatment for all NHS patients who wanted it.

Careful stimulation and monitoring in intrauterine insemination cycles should reduce the risks of too many follicles developing. If this does occur then it may be appropriate to convert the cycle to in vitro fertilisation, where all the eggs are retrieved, or cancel the cycle without the administration of human chorionic gonadotrophin. Nevertheless, patients whose insemination cycle is abandoned should be counselled about the persistent risk of spontaneous pregnancy and advised to use condoms during intercourse for the rest of the cycle.

However, because it is common practice to transfer more than one embryo, in vitro fertilisation and intracytoplasmic sperm injection cycles often result in twin or triplet pregnancies. In the United Kingdom under the terms of the Human Fertilisation and Embryology Authority (HFEA) code of practice, no more than two embryos may be transferred in a treatment cycle—except in special circumstances, when three may be used. With continuing improvements in cryopreservation and embryo culture there are moves to encourage the transfer of only one embryo at a time.

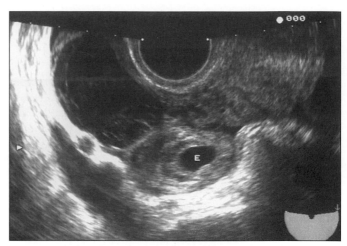
Ectopic pregnancy diagnosed using ultrasonography

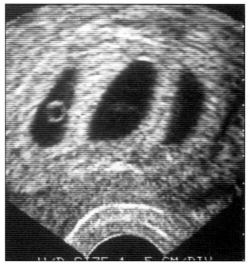
Ultrasound picture of an early triplet pregnancy

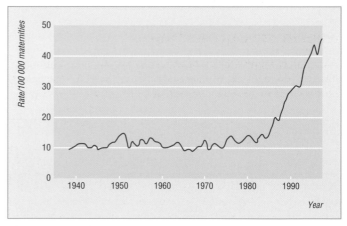
Triplet and other higher order births in England and Wales, 1938-97

Advantages of embryo cryopreservation

- Maximises conception potential from an in vitro fertilisation or intracytoplasmic sperm injection stimulation cycle
- Prevents wastage of any surplus embryos
- Allows embryo transfer in a natural cycle with no risk of OHSS
- Reduces the cost of treatment as gonadotrophins are not needed
- No need for women receiving oocyte donation to synchronise their cycle with the donor

Creation of surplus embryos

Under the terms of the HFEA code of practice, patients having assisted conception may not have more than three embryos transferred in any vitro fertilisation, intracytoplasmic sperm injection, or frozen cycle. Usually only two embryos are transferred unless there are cogent clinical reasons. With the use of superovulation and increasingly successful techniques to achieve fertilisation in vitro, more than three embryos are often available at the time of transfer, giving couples certain choices for the embryos not transferred immediately.

The surplus embryos can be frozen so that they are available for use in a subsequent cycle. Cryopreservation of gametes or embryos requires a stepwise exposure to cryoprotectants, cooling to subzero temperatures, and storage in liquid nitrogen at − 196°C. The embryos can remain in storage without deterioration until they are needed for use in treatment by means of thawing, rehydration, and removal of the cryoprotectant. Not all embryos are suitable for cryopreservation. Only around two thirds of embryos will survive the freezing and thawing process, and survival will depend mainly on the quality (cleavage stage and morphology) of the embryos.

When embryos are unsuitable for freezing, or if couples are concerned about cryopreservation they may choose to allow them to perish, or they can donate them to research projects approved by the HFEA. Details of these projects can be found on the HFEA's website (www.hfea.gov.uk).

Couples should receive counselling on all the options before starting a cycle, which will give them time to consider their choices. Their wishes must be recorded on a form from the HFEA, signed copies of which are retained in their notes and by the individuals concerned.

Variable success of implantation and pregnancy rates with frozen thawed embryos has been reported. The rates range from 10% live birth rate to rates equivalent to those achieved with fresh embryos. The success of the freeze-thaw process and subsequent transfer can depend on the clinic where it is done. The success rates for various clinics can be seen on the HFEA's website (www.hfea.gov.uk/ForPatients).

Sperm cryopreservation

Although cryopreservation of semen from animals and humans has been done for many years, and refinements of the technology have allowed increases in the yield of motile sperm surviving,

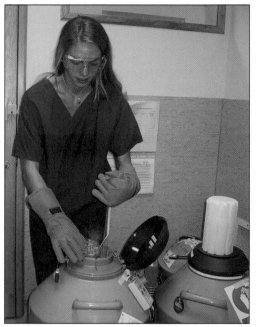

Straw containing frozen embryos being removed from liquid nitrogen storage dewar for thawing before embryo transfer

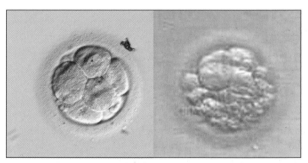

Two eight-cell embryos of different quality. Left: high quality. Right: low quality

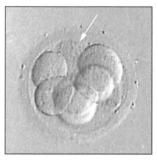

Thawed embryo with six out of eight cells surviving the freeze-thaw process. The outlines of the two lysed cells are visible (arrow)

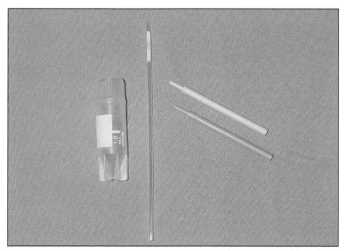

Plasticware and colour coders used in cryopreservation of semen and embryos

---

Uses of sperm cryopreservation

- For donor insemination cycles
- To store sperm before chemotherapy or radiotherapy to preserve the man's fertility potential
- To avoid the need for repeat surgery by freezing sperm that are surgically retrieved
- To store sperm for a treatment cycle if difficulty in producing a sperm sample is anticipated

fresh samples are still about 30% better in quality than frozen samples. In the past, poor quality semen samples may have been discarded as unsuitable for treatment, but intracytoplasmic sperm injection has made it worth cryopreserving any sample that contains some live, motile sperm.

When to stop treatment

It is difficult for both patient and clinician to decide when to stop treatment. On the basis of the couple's history, the clinician will advise them on their prognosis. The couple can then make a decision whether to stop treatment. Clinicians rarely have to advise patients to stop treatment because the stress of the repeated procedures, physically and mentally, usually leads the couple to reach the appropriate decision. However, a pregnancy, even if it results in an early pregnancy loss, may give encouragement to the couple and make it more difficult for them to decide to stop treatment. Repeated failed cycles (despite good quality embryos) are uncommon, but when they do occur the couple can feel frustrated and vulnerable. These emotions may encourage them to shop from clinic to clinic, hoping that some new treatment (for example, assisted hatching, aneuploidy screening, miscarriage treatment) may be offered to enable them to become pregnant.

Usually, the circumstances are clearer when few or poor quality oocytes are produced, even with high doses of gonadotrophins. Generally, this reflects a decline in the number of oocytes in the ovary (decreased ovarian reserve). This decline happens naturally as women age, but may occur surprisingly early in some women. These women may have normal cycles, but could have incipient ovarian failure, which makes it harder for them to understand their failure to conceive and to come to terms with their premature childlessness. Oocyte donation is their only way of conception; adoption is another approach. Exit counselling is important and helpful in these circumstances.

Competing interests: None declared.

Further reading

- Royal College of Obstetricians and Gynaecologists. *Evidence-based guidelines: initial investigation and management of the infertile couple.* London: RCOG, 1998
- Templeton A, Ashok P, Bhattacharya S, Gazvani R, Hamilton M, Macmillan S, et al. *Management of infertility for the MRCOG and beyond.* London: RCOG, 2000
- Balen AH, Jacobs HS. *Infertility in practice.* London: Churchhill Livingstone, 1997
- Mortimer D. *Practical laboratory andrology.* Oxford: Oxford University Press, 1994
- Meniru GI, Brinsden PR, Craft I, eds. *A handbook of intrauterine insemination.* Cambridge: Cambridge University Press, 1997
- Code of Practice. 5th ed. www.hfea.gov.uk/HFEAPublications

10 Assisted conception and the law in the United Kingdom

Peter Braude, Sadia Muhammed

Along with advances in technology comes the need for government guidelines and laws to ensure that those technologies are used safely and responsibly. This article covers the development of the rules in the United Kingdom that govern assisted conception, and the implications of these rules for day to day clinical practice.

Human Fertilisation and Embryology Act 1990

The Human Fertilisation and Embryology Act was passed in 1990 in response to the report of the Committee of Inquiry into Human Fertilisation and Embryology (the Warnock report), which examined three main public concerns. These were:

● Creation of human embryos outside the body and their use in treatment
● Use of human embryos in research
● Use of donated gametes and embryos.

The act established the Human Fertilisation and Embryology Authority (HFEA), and its licensing and inspection procedures, as the main mechanism for regulating these activities.

Functions of the HFEA

The HFEA is a statutory non-departmental public body and is accountable to the secretary of state for health. Established in 1991, it is the first statutory body of its type in the world. It has 18 members who are appointed by the secretary of state, including a lay chairperson and a deputy chairperson. At least one third, but not more than half, of its membership may be registered medical practitioners or those who have been involved with assisted conception or its research funding.

Licensing

Three types of licences can be granted by the HFEA.

A *treatment licence* allows the unit to pursue treatments that fall under the act.

A *storage licence* allows cryopreservation and storage of gametes and embryos.

A *research licence* is needed to perform any research that uses human embryos in vitro.

To practise assisted conception, the centre will be inspected and, if the facilities and staff are deemed suitable, a treatment licence will be granted to the "person responsible." This person will be the named individual under whose supervision the licensed activities will be carried out. In the United Kingdom certain activities are prohibited and a breach of the act is considered a criminal offence. The renewable licence is granted for up to three years, but is subject to annual reports and inspections.

The register

The act requires the HFEA to keep a register of all treatment cycles and of all children born as a result of in vitro fertilisation

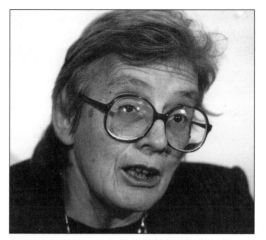

Baroness Mary Warnock chaired the Committee of Inquiry into Human Fertilisation and Embryology 1982-4

Assisted conception treatments that require an HFEA licence*

● In vitro fertilisation
● Intracytoplasmic sperm injection
● Preimplantation genetic diagnosis
● Sperm donation
● Egg donation
● Embryo donation
● Surrogacy

*Other assisted conception treatments, such as intrauterine insemination and gamete intrafallopian transfer, do not need a licence if own gametes are used as no embryo is created in vitro

---

Research using human embryos in vitro permitted under an HFEA research licence

● To promote advances in the treatment of infertility
● To increase knowledge about the causes of congenital disease
● To increase knowledge about the causes of miscarriage
● To develop more effective techniques of contraception
● To develop methods for detecting the presence of gene or chromosome abnormalities in embryos before implantation
● To increase knowledge about the development of embryos*
● To increase knowledge about serious disease*
● To enable any such knowledge to be applied in developing treatments for serious disease*
● To enable any such knowledge to be applied in developing treatments for serious disease*

*Added in 2001 after the parliamentary debate on use of embryos for the creation of stem cells (Human Fertilisation and Embryology (Research Purposes) Regulations)

Activities prohibited in the act

● Keeping or using an embryo in vitro after the appearance of the primitive streak or 14 days of development, whichever is the earlier
● Placing an embryo in a non-human animal
● Replacing the nucleus of an embryo with a nucleus taken from the cells of another person or another embryo (cloning)
● Altering the genetic structure of any cell while it forms part of an embryo

---

technology or by the use of donated eggs or sperm. The register ensures that later on such children may learn something of the circumstances of their conception. The act states that when children reach 18 years they may request to know whether they were born as a result of a treatment that required an HFEA licence, including donor insemination. If contemplating marriage, the child may ask whether they could be related to the individual that they intend to marry. In these circumstances, the request may be made by a minor of marriageable age, and so the first such requests for information may be expected in 2007 (16 years after the establishment of the HFEA). Under current legislation the identity of donors will not be revealed.

Implications of the act for practice

The HFEA publishes and revises regularly its code of practice in which is set out what are considered "suitable practices" in the context of activities that require licences under the act. The act is unusual in clinical practice in five principal ways.

Consent

The act requires that control of the use of gametes, whether for in vitro fertilisation, storage, donation, or research should lie with the provider of those gametes (but without the notion of ownership). Consent forms are used to specify the fate of embryos and gametes in assisted conception.

It is this requirement for written consent that was at the heart of the dispute in the case of Diane Blood. While he lay in a coma, Diane Blood wanted some of her husband's sperm removed to be cryopreserved for her later use to have a child. Removal and storage of the sperm and its use without written consent would have been a criminal offence in the United Kingdom. After a protracted court case Diane Blood was allowed to take the sperm abroad for use.

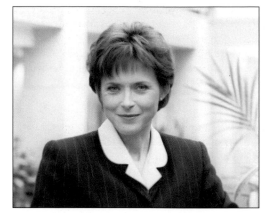

Suzi Leather chairs the HFEA

Other functions of the HFEA

- To publicise the services provided by the HFEA or provided in the pursuance of licences. This is done through the HFEA's annual report and website (www.hfea.gov.uk)
- To provide advice and information to those to whom licences apply and to those who are receiving treatment, providing gametes or embryos, or who may wish to do so (guides and leaflets for patients)
- To keep under review information about embryos and about the provision of treatment services, and (when asked) to advise the secretary of state on such matters

---

Activities that consent must specify

- The precise use of the gametes in treatment
- Whether gametes may be used to fertilise an egg in vitro and whose eggs may be fertilised
- Into whom those embryos may be placed
- What is to be done with any embryos not transferred (they could be frozen, destroyed, or used for research)
- Whether any embryos or gametes may be cryopreserved, and if so then the length of time for which they may be stored
- The precise use of those cryopreserved gametes or embryos including their use after the death of the donors involved

Confidentiality

Because of the sensitive and personal nature of the treatments involved, specific criminal sanctions exist for a breach of confidentiality. It is unusual for confidentiality to be enforced so strictly, and even more so that criminal sanctions can be brought if broken. In practice, assisted conception unit case notes are kept securely and separately from routine hospital notes. They are accessible only to those members of the unit named on the treatment licence, or when needed, to other licensed individuals. An amendment to the act in 1992 allowed information about the treatment to be given to a third party only with the patient's explicit written consent and strictly on a "need to know" basis.

Counselling

Before providing or receiving gametes for use, donation, or fertilisation, the act requires that a person must have "a suitable opportunity to receive proper counselling on the implications of taking the proposed steps," and that that their consent should

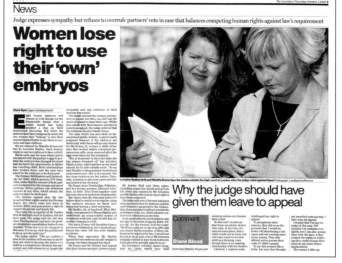

Lorraine Hadley and Natallie Evans separated from their partners with whom they had had IVF treatment and embryos frozen. The men withdrew their consent, however, and the embryos must now be destroyed. The High Court in London upheld the ruling that effective consent must be given by both the man and the woman to allow continued storage of their embryos

General practitioners may find that, because of the strict confidentiality of the Human Fertilisation and Embryology Act, summaries and information about the assisted conception treatment that their patient is having may not be forthcoming if that is their patient's wish. Sometimes letters from the unit will be sent to the patient for them to release to their doctor as they see fit

not be effective unless such counselling has been offered. All reproductive medicine units should provide access to an appropriately trained fertility counsellor, although the patients do not have to accept the offer of counselling to receive treatment. Counselling for people having treatment in which donor gametes are to be used is strongly advised.

Information
The act also requires that no person should provide gametes for in vitro fertilisation, storage, or donation without first being given appropriate information about treatment. All assisted conception units are therefore obliged to have written information available (including up to date success rates expressed as "live birth per treatment cycle started"), which can be requested by prospective patients or their doctors. The HFEA patients' guides also have information about these success rates, including multiple pregnancy rates and services offered at the 110 units that hold treatment licences in the United Kingdom. The patients' guides and other publications can be obtained free from the HFEA, Paxton House, 30 Artillery Lane, London E1 7LS.

Welfare of the child
The welfare of the child is probably the most controversial part of the act. It requires that "a woman shall not be provided with treatment services unless account has been taken of the welfare of any child who may be born as a result of the treatment (including the need of that child for a father) and of any other child who may be affected by the birth." The latter refers to any existing children in the family

Thus, each licensed unit is obliged to have clear written procedures for assessing the welfare of the potential child and of any other child who may be affected. However, this condition applies only to centres that hold a treatment licence. It has been argued that this requirement is unfair because it does not apply to natural procreation, nor does it apply to fertility treatments offered outside licensed assisted conception units.

Nevertheless all assisted conception units should ask the couple's general practitioner for information about any factors that may be relevant to the couple's suitability as parents of the child. Permission from the patient is usually included in the letter of request from the unit.

Some units may provide helpful checklists to ensure that they ask about specific issues that are deemed relevant. These issues include whether the couple live together, whether any of their children have been put on the "at risk" register or taken into care, and whether either partner has a drug dependence, a history of violence, or a criminal record. After assessment, if a unit decides that it cannot treat the couple, the couple concerned must be told, and they may then appeal against this decision or seek treatment at another unit.

> **Providing information about a patient's suitability to be a parent may be regarded as intrusive and hence the general practitioner should ensure that he or she has specific permission from the patient**

Legal parents of children from donated gametes or surrogacy

The woman's husband will be the legal father of a child born using donated sperm unless they are judicially separated or he can prove that he did not consent to the treatment. Where a

---

Additional information a centre requires when providing treatment with donor gametes
- A child's potential need to know about his or her origins and whether the prospective parents are prepared for the question if it arises as the child is growing up
- The possible attitudes of other members of the family towards the child and the child's status in the family
- The implication for the welfare of the child if the donor is personally known in the child's family and social circle
- Any possibility known to the centre of a dispute about the legal fatherhood of the child

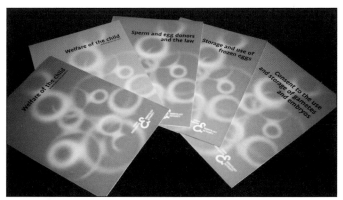

Patients' guides available from the HFEA

Information to be taken into account when assessing welfare of the child issues
- The couple's commitment to having and bringing up a child or children
- The couple's ability to provide a stable and supportive environment for any child produced as result of treatment
- The couple's medical histories and the histories of their families
- The couple's health and consequent future ability to look after or provide for a child's needs
- The couple's ages and their likely future ability to look after or provide for a child's needs
- The couple's ability to meet the needs of any child, including children in multiple births
- Any risk of harm to the child or children who may be born, including the risk of inherited disorders, transmissible diseases, or problems of neglect or abuse
- The effect of a new baby or babies on any existing child of the family

---

Transfer of legal parentage to a commissioning couple in a surrogacy arrangement
- The child must be genetically related to at least one member of the commissioning couple
- The surrogate parents must have consented to the making of the parental order for transfer no earlier than six weeks after the birth of the child
- The commissioning couple must have applied for a parental order within six months of the child's birth
- The commissioning couple must be married to each other and both be over 18 years
- No money other than expenses must have been paid in respect of the surrogacy arrangement unless authorised by a court
- The child must be living with the commissioning couple
- The commissioning couple must be domiciled in the United Kingdom, the Channel Islands, or the Isle of Man

woman is being treated together with a male partner who is not her husband and uses donated sperm, and if her legal husband does not consent to the treatment, then that male partner will be the legal father of any resulting child. Consent forms will normally reflect this intent.

When a woman receives donated oocytes, she, as the "birth mother" is the legal mother of the child, and her partner or husband is the legal father.

Surrogacy is a special case, and the child has to be adopted formally even though it is genetically derived from one or both parents. The birth mother and her partner are the legal parents of a child born as a result of a surrogacy arrangement until legal parentage is transferred to the commissioning couple. The surrogate mother must therefore register the baby to whom she has given birth in the normal way. Her husband or partner should normally be registered as the father. Surrogacy arrangements between the commissioning couple and the surrogate mother are not legally enforceable under UK law, even when the child results from an embryo created from the gametes of the commissioning couple.

The photograph of Mary Warnock is reproduced with permission from the Press Association and the photograph of Suzi Leather is reproduced with permission from the HFEA. The *Guardian* page is the 2 October 2003 issue.

Competing interests: None declared.

Regulations in the United States

- No federal law exists to govern the practice of assisted conception in the United States except for the requirement of the 1992 Fertility Clinic Success Rate and Certification Act for each in vitro fertilisation or intracytoplasmic sperm injection programme to report annually its pregnancy success rates to the United States Centers for Disease Control and Prevention (CDC)
- These data are analysed and published as the Assisted Reproductive Technology Report by the CDC in conjunction with the Society of Assisted Reproductive Technology (SART)
- The report can be found at www.cdc.gov/reproductivehealth/ART00/index.htm
- Minimum standard practice guidelines are issued by the American Society of Reproductive Medicine, which are updated periodically (www.asrm.org)

Further reading

- *The Human Fertilisation and Embryology Act.* London: HMSO, 1990
- *The Surrogacy Arrangements Act.* London: HMSO, 1985
- Morgan D, Lee R. *Blackstone's guide to the Human Fertilisation and Embryology Act.* London: Blackstone Press, 2001
- Gunning J, ed. *Assisted conception: research ethics and the law.* Aldershot: Ashgate Publishing, 2000
- Warnock M. *An intelligent person's guide to ethics.* London: George Duckworth, 1998

11 Counselling

Alison Bagshawe, Alison Taylor

Subfertility usually affects a person's capacity to function normally in close personal relationships, socially, and at work. Many couples find that facing the problem of subfertility, and coping with the investigations and treatments can cause anxiety, stress, and depression. Demands and pressures may be placed on subfertile couples by different cultural, religious, and familial attitudes towards parenthood and childlessness. These factors can also affect the way each individual feels about and responds to the problem.

Subfertility and couples' relationships

Tensions and conflicts within close relationships are common, and many couples experience a degree of sexual dysfunction in their attempts to conceive. A history of termination of pregnancy, recurrent miscarriages, sexually transmitted infections, or sterilisation can all become a source of conflict. One or both partners may feel guilty or a have sense of failure, and as a result misunderstandings and blame can occur, which may cause the breakdown of relationships. Men and women usually experience subfertility and its treatment in different ways, and lengthy treatments may have an impact on work and on domestic and social lives.

The role of the counsellor

Opening up clearer communication
The counsellor's task is to deal with the stress of the situation by exploring what has led to it, and to help find ways of opening up clearer communication between partners. Advice is not given on how the situation should be resolved, but instead the counsellor asks the couple what they would like to change and helps them explore how each of them might do this.

Counselling aims to clarify the needs arising from the impact of fertility problems on the person's emotional, psychological, and social life. Supporting and encouraging the expression of difficult feelings and emotions can help that person to adjust to their circumstances and relate to their environment in a more constructive way.

How much counselling?
The frequency, duration, and focus of counselling varies and will depend on the circumstances of the couple. One hour may be enough for some couples; others will need several sessions. Important objectives of counselling include encouraging people to clarify the underlying nature of a problem or difficulty, and exploring the capacity that the couple has to deal with the problem.

Counselling and fertility treatment
Couples often have conflicting thoughts and feelings about a proposed form of treatment. Being given the opportunity to discuss the different options available and the implications of any proposed treatment can help them reach an informed decision that is acceptable to both partners. Adequate preparation through counselling before treatment can substantially decrease the "roller coaster" effect to which many couples have likened the experience of infertility treatment.

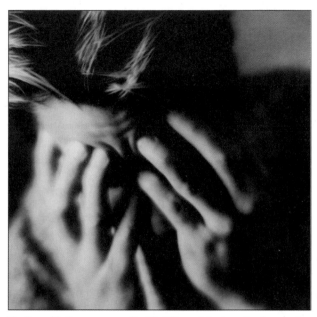

Dealing with the pressures of subfertility and the investigations and treatments can cause anxiety, stress, and depression

Counselling does not offer medical or clinical judgments, opinions, or decisions

Counselling for patients who want to store, discard, or offer for research or donation excess embryos from an in vitro fertilisation cycle will focus on the legal, moral, and ethical dilemmas that may concern some people about these options

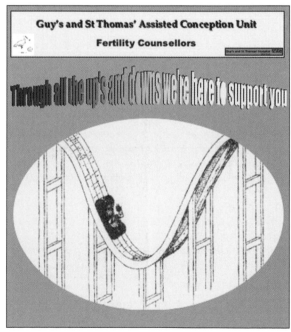

Counselling may help reduce the "roller coaster" effect of infertility treatment

Expectations of reproductive technologies are often too high and, where treatment is unsuccessful, personal inadequacy and a sense of failure leave many feeling emotionally exhausted and vulnerable.

Legal requirements

Under the terms of the UK 1990 Human Fertilisation and Embryology Act and as stated in the Human Fertilisation and Embryology Authority's code of practice, people seeking licensed treatment must be given the opportunity to receive counselling before consenting to treatment.

Types of counselling

Three types of counselling are recognised.

Implications counselling explores with the person how any proposed treatment would affect them, their family, and any child born as a result of treatment. Although genetic counselling falls into this category, this type of counselling is of a different style and nature to general counselling. Donors in particular must consider the short and long term effects that any donation could have on a future child, existing children, and the family as a whole. In addition, recipients of donated gametes must consider the rights of a future child to information about his or her genetic origins.

Support counselling aims to give emotional support at any time before, during, or after treatment. This may mean providing a support group or offering assistance to find a suitable one.

Therapeutic counselling focuses on the effects, consequences, and resolution of treatment and infertility. Referral to someone who can give longer term or more appropriate therapeutic counselling should be offered if necessary.

The welfare of the child

The Human Fertilisation and Embryology Act requires that before any treatment is given at a licensed centre certain welfare issues must be taken into consideration: the welfare of any child born as a result of treatment; the need of that child for a father; and the needs of any existing child who may be affected by the birth.

Assessing the welfare of the child

Many factors must be considered in this assessment, including who would be legally responsible for any child and who intends to bring up the child. The act does not exclude any category of woman from being considered for treatment. However, in situations where the child would have no legal father, the centre must pay particular attention to the prospective mother's ability to meet the child's needs throughout childhood. This includes considering other members in the family or social group of the woman who might share this responsibility and who might act as male role models.

Assessment includes taking a detailed medical and social history. Consideration is given to other areas, such as the degree of commitment to having a child and the ability to provide a stable and supportive environment. In addition, the age, health, and medical history of the potential parents are important. Any risk of harm to the future child, including the risk of inherited disorders, transmittable disease, problems during pregnancy, and the implications of multiple birth must be considered. Possible neglect or abuse in the future and the effects that either the treatment or a new baby would have on any existing children must be taken into account.

> **Although recognised as beneficial, counselling is not mandatory. However, it is common practice for clinics to make it a requirement of treatment for couples seeking use of donor gametes or embryos or for treatments such as surrogacy**

Support groups for patients

- UK National Fertility Association (ISSUE) 01922 722888 (www.issue.co.uk)
- The National Infertility Support Network (CHILD) 01424 732361 (www.child.org.uk)
- Donor Conception Network 020 8245 4369 (dcnetwork.org)
- Daisy Network (www.daisynetwork.org.uk)
- HFEA (www.hfea.gov.uk)

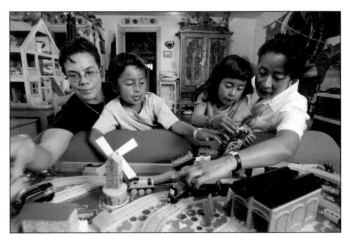

When assessing the welfare of the child, factors such as who will bring up the child are taken into consideration. Reproduced with permission of Eric Risberg/AP

Role of the general practitioner

- Reproductive medicine centres must be satisfied that the general practitioner of each prospective parent knows of no reason why either may not be suitable for the treatment to be offered
- General practitioners are asked to provide factual information, medical or otherwise, that might have implications for the health or welfare of any resulting child
- Before general practitioners are asked for information about patients, written consent is sought from their patient, and failure to give this consent is taken into account when the clinic considers whether to offer treatment

---

Assessment protocol

Assessment of a couple seeking treatment takes place according to a protocol set up by each reproductive medicine unit. Questionnaires are usually used and are completed by the patients and their general practitioners. Information gained at the initial consultation is also included. Where concerns are raised, further investigation and assessment may be needed before a decision can be made about whether treatment should be offered.

Role of the counsellor in assessment

Sometimes the counsellor may play a role in the assessment (although this process is at odds with the usual client-counsellor relationship), and the purpose of the session must be made clear to the couple being seen. The limits of confidentiality must also be specified at the start of a session, as some information may need to be shared with the clinical team before a decision to treat or not can be made. If the counsellor takes part in the assessment process in this way, patients should have access to an alternative independent counsellor for supportive and therapeutic counselling. If there is difficulty in making a decision, cases may be referred to an ethics committee.

Refusal of treatment

Treatment may be refused by the centre on clinical grounds or if the centre believes that it would not be in the best interests of any resulting or existing child. Treatment may also be withheld if there is not enough information or advice to allow a decision to be made. If treatment is denied, the centre must explain their reasons, offer the couple options that remain open, and say where counselling can be obtained.

Competing interests: None declared.

Key points

- Subfertility (and dealing with the investigations and treatments) can cause anxiety, stress, and depression
- Counselling aims to help people identify the needs arising from the impact of subfertility on their emotional, psychological, and social life
- Counselling can reduce the roller coaster effect of treatment
- Three types of counselling are recognised: implications counselling, support counselling, and therapeutic counselling
- Licensed centres must offer patients access to counselling
- Licensed centres must assess the welfare of any child born as a result of treatment, the need of that child for a father, and the needs of any existing children who may be affected by the birth

Further reading

- Read J. *Counselling for fertility problems.* London: Sage, 1995
- Campion MJ, ed. *Who's fit to be a parent?* London: Routledge, 1995
- Human Fertilisation and Embryology Authority code of practice. www.hfea.gov.uk

12   Intractable infertility

Alison Bagshawe, Alison Taylor

It is rare for any of the options available for couples with intractable infertility to be seen as a first choice. For many couples in this situation infertility is like bereavement and causes great emotional distress. However, with help, people may be able to accept their position and see the opportunity to start a new life. To embrace any of the following options and to cope with the complications and frustrations of each, psychological strength and stamina are needed, plus help from a skilled independent counsellor.

Egg, sperm, and embryo donation

Counselling for gamete and embryo donation
Counselling for those receiving donor gametes or embryos encourages them to explore concerns and feelings related to their infertility before considering the social and emotional issues that may arise from non-genetic parenthood. The emotional impact and implications of donation can cause problems for recipients. Men and women often have different thoughts and feelings about the donors and about accepting donated gametes or embryos.

Short and long term implications of donation are influenced by the attitude, beliefs, and personal and social situation of the individuals concerned. Sperm, egg, and embryo donation can be from an anonymous or a known donor, and each has different implications. Counselling can be relatively straightforward or complex depending on the circumstances, and the counselling sessions will vary in length and intensity accordingly. Counselling explores the implications of a person's reasoning and challenges their assumptions and preconceptions. Issues such as openness or secrecy must be considered, as well as the questions of whether to tell the potential future child about their genetic background, and what, how, and when to tell both the child and the wider family.

Selection and screening of donors
Information is given about the selection and screening of donors. Gamete donors have to give a detailed personal, medical, family, and genetic history and are screened for sexually transmitted infections including HIV, hepatitis B and C, and other viral infections, such as cytomegalovirus. Their karyotype is checked and they are offered counselling before they consent to donate their gametes. Donors are invited to write non-identifying information about themselves that can be made available to recipients.

Quarantining donated semen
Sperm quality is assessed and, if initial screening tests are normal, semen is frozen. Samples remain quarantined for six months, at which point an HIV test is repeated (to exclude recently acquired infection before seroconversion). If all results are negative, samples can then be released for clinical use. Egg donation is usually with fresh eggs rather than frozen eggs because it is more difficult to freeze eggs than sperm. Recipients need to be aware of the small potential risk of HIV transmission from a donor who has recently acquired the infection but not yet become seropositive.

Options for intractable infertility
- Egg, sperm, or embryo donation
- Adoption
- Surrogacy
- Accepting a childless lifestyle

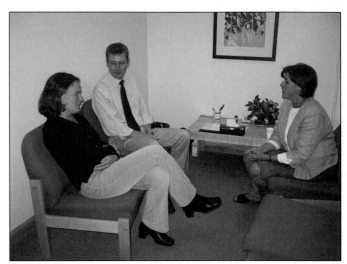

For many couples, facing the situation of intractable infertility is extremely distressing and help from a counsellor may be needed

---

Issues explored in counselling for couples pursuing gamete or embryo donation
- Concerns and emotions associated with infertility and non-genetic parenthood
- Various implications of gamete or embryo donation depending on the couple's cultural, religious, and moral beliefs
- Selection, screening, and legal status of donors and recipients
- Whether, what, when, and how to tell a child about his or her genetic background and what, when, and how to tell the wider family

---

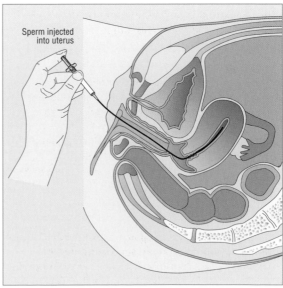

Donor insemination

Legal issues

The legal status of the donor, recipient, and future child should be discussed as part of counselling before treatment. Under the terms of the UK 1990 Human Fertilisation and Embryology Act, the woman giving birth to the child is the legal mother, and her husband or partner is the legal father (unless he can show he did not consent to treatment), irrespective of whether gametes or embryos used were their own or donated.

As the law currently stands, donor anonymity is protected, although the child has the right to contact the Human Fertilisation and Embryology Authority at 18 years (or 16 years if wishing to marry) to ask if he or she was born as a result of gamete donation and if a prospective partner might be related. However, a revision of law is being considered that may in future allow the identity of donors to be known, and recipients should be encouraged to consider how they might feel about the right of a child to this information.

Adoption

As a result of the UK 1980 Children Act the "welfare of the child" is paramount. Most adoption agreements support "open adoption," which encourages honesty with the child and ongoing links with the birth family. Recruitment and placing is often made with a particular child in mind, and preliminary assessments try to ensure a match between the child and the potential parents.

Adoption after infertility treatment

A couple who have been trying to conceive their own child must change their perspective before adoption can be considered seriously. Coming to terms with infertility before embarking on this option is essential. Counselling aims to help this process and to prepare the couple for the reality of adoption.

Adoption agencies and the assessment process

All adoptions must be through an adoption agency, either local authority or voluntary, and each has its own criteria for adoption. Interviews take place over several months before a child is placed. Issues such as the couple's attitudes to their infertility and their motives for wanting to adopt will be explored exhaustively to assess the couple's stability and commitment to adoption. The process can be lengthy, and counsellors who do not take part in the assessment can offer support, a fresh perspective, and a safe environment in which the couple can explore their thoughts and feelings.

Overseas adoption

Adoption from overseas can be complex and expensive, although some countries have reciprocal arrangements with the United Kingdom. However, political or legal idiosyncrasies and differing attitudes to adoption can make this a difficult course to follow. A "home study" report carried out through an adoption agency is needed, and applications to adopt a child must be approved by the Home Office and local social services.

Surrogacy

In surrogacy, one woman (the surrogate or host mother) carries a child for another as the result of an agreement (before conception) that the child should be handed over after birth. The couple wishing to bring up the child after the birth is the commissioning couple.

> **Donors do not have any parental rights or responsibilities towards any children born after treatment and can withdraw consent to the use of gametes or embryos up to the point of transfer to a recipient**

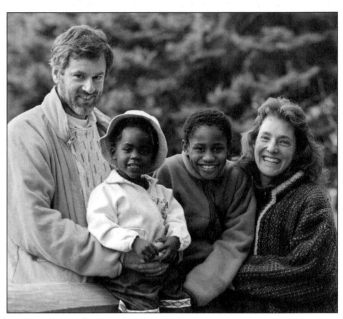

Overseas adoption can be difficult and expensive

Overseas adoption support groups for patients

- Overseas Adoption Helpline
  64-66 High Street
  Barnet
  Herts EN5 5SJ
  0870 516 8742 (www.oah.org.uk)
- Overseas Adoption Support and Information Service (OASIS)
  20 Woodland Terrace
  Green Bank
  Plymouth PL4 8NL
  0870 241 7069 (www.adoptionoverseas.org)

Types of surrogacy arrangement

Partial surrogacy—The woman who carries the child (host mother) also provides the egg and is therefore the genetic mother of the child. Partial surrogacy can be achieved by donor insemination, home insemination, or as a result of in vitro fertilisation treatment

Full surrogacy—The host mother is not genetically related to the child but has embryos donated by the commissioning couple. Alternatively, embryos may have resulted from a known or anonymous donation to the commissioning couple. Full surrogacy can be achieved only through an in vitro fertilisation cycle undergone by the woman (or donor) of the commissioning couple

Legal issues

In the United Kingdom, surrogacy agreements between the surrogate and commissioning couple are not enforceable legally. The law allows parents of children born after gamete donation to be the legal parents of the resulting child or children at birth. This means the surrogate mother can be regarded as having received donated gametes to conceive. She is therefore the legal mother of the resulting child at birth. The commissioning couple have to apply through the courts to become the legal parents of the child or children. Hence, there is difficulty enforcing a surrogacy arrangement if the surrogate changes her mind and feels unable to give up the child to the commissioning couple.

Counselling for surrogacy

Counselling for surrogacy is lengthy and comprehensive. Home visits and several appointments are often needed. All concerned must understand the implications of what is intended and they must be committed to the proposed arrangements. The underlying focus of counselling should be to protect any existing and future child or children, as well as any adults who are involved, from possible distress and complications that could result from an ill informed or ill considered decision.

Accepting a child-free lifestyle

For some couples, letting go and moving on from treatment is a relief, whereas for others it is a traumatic experience. Acceptance of a child-free lifestyle only comes over time, and often after great psychological and emotional adjustment. Choosing a child-free life is totally different from being forced into childlessness through circumstance. Those facing this possibility often ask how others come to accept it, but there is no simple answer.

Experiences from childhood of what parenting is, and how positive or negative it is seen to be, can build or destroy an individual's sense of self. Infertility and subsequent treatment can erode a person's confidence. Positive experiences from childhood therefore help people to cope more constructively with childlessness.

Support from partners, friends, and family is vital for couples coming to terms with infertility and accepting a child-free lifestyle. Cultural, religious, and social factors that determine a couple's attitudes to the value of children and their importance to family life can either help or hinder. It is easier for those whose family and wider social group accept childlessness to live with and adapt to a life without children than it is for those whose culture places more importance on the need for children in family life.

Counselling

Counselling for people who are trying to accept a childless future varies in frequency and intensity, and, if offered appropriately, it can be therapeutic and supportive. A person trying to accept a child-free lifestyle may visit their general practitioner with symptoms such as repetitive minor ailments, minor gynaecological problems, depression, loss of appetite, sleeplessness, and conflict in relationships. Recognising the underlying reasons for their symptoms and offering appropriate intervention at this stage can help and lead to the beginning of acceptance. Feelings of depression, being "stuck," and hopelessness are common, and, until these are dealt with adequately, they will impede a person's ability to see any point to the future. Looking ahead to other changes and recognising that a future can exist without children gives a focus for counselling that mobilises the coping strategies of each person.

Issues explored in counselling for surrogacy

- The law relating to surrogacy arrangements
- Treatment including the risks, multiple birth, termination and failure of treatment or pregnancy, and possible disability of a child
- Existing children—what they know, how they will be prepared, what arrangements have been made, and how parents will deal with concerns such as attachment, loss, separation, anxiety, and jealousy
- The unborn child, including managing a pregnancy, complications, and the future needs of the child
- Relationships with family, friends, colleagues, and their attitudes, expectations, and hopes
- Practicalities of the birth—bonding, breast feeding, handing over the baby, and future contact

---

Surrogacy support groups for patients

- Childlessness Overcome Through Surrogacy (COTS)
  Lairg
  Sutherland IV27 4EF
  0844 414 0181 (www.surrogacy.org.uk)
- Surrogacy UK
  01531 821889—Carol O'Reilly
  (www.surrogacyuk.org)

Before a child-free life is accepted, the grief and loss experienced may cause a person to visit their general practitioner with repetitive minor health problems, depression, and conflict in relationships

---

Further reading

- Blythe E, Crawshaw M, Spiers J, eds. *Truth and the child 10 years on: information exchange in donor assisted conception.* Birmingham: British Association of Social Workers, 1998
- Snowden R, Snowden EM. *The gift of a child.* Exeter: Exeter University Press, 1993
- Stanton AL, Dunkel-Scheffer C. *Infertility perspectives from stress and coping research.* New York: Plenum Press, 1991
- Mason MC. *Male infertility—men talking.* London: Routledge, 1993
- Humphrey M, Humphrey H. *Families with a difference—varieties of surrogate parenthood.* London: Routledge, 1998

The photograph of a family with adopted children is reproduced with permission of Nancy Palmieri/AP.

Competing interests: None declared.

13   Further advances and uses of assisted conception technology

Susan Pickering, Peter Braude

Assisted conception technology has led to a variety of new techniques that can help subfertile couples. However, many now go beyond simply improving the capacity to procreate. They also affect areas outside reproductive biology and present new ethical dilemmas.

Preserving fertility for young women

Long term survival rates for cancer have improved substantially because of the use of aggressive chemotherapy and radiotherapy. However, in young women this comes at a price—many women lose ovarian function because oocytes or their support cells are damaged by the treatment. A technique ensuring successful cryopreservation of oocytes would benefit women recently diagnosed with cancer who want to retain their fertility potential. In addition, cryopreservation could help women with a family history of premature menopause as they could store their gametes before their pool of oocytes is depleted.

Cryopreservation of oocytes
In contrast to the success of embryo freezing, which is now a routine procedure in most in vitro fertilisation clinics, cryopreservation of oocytes has been less successful. Only a few live births after egg freezing have been achieved since the first one in 1986. Some problems have been reduced by improving cryoprotectant regimens and by using intracytoplasmic sperm injection to overcome the block to fertilisation, resulting in a few pregnancies and live births. However, the success rate remains low—about 1 in 100 eggs that are frozen results in a live birth.

Cryopreservation of ovarian tissue and maturation of oocytes and follicles in vitro
An alternative approach is cryopreservation of slices or biopsies of ovarian tissue, which contain many thousands of immature oocytes. These oocytes are quiescent and their chromatin is in a stable phase of meiosis.

Autografting and in vitro maturation could be used to recover frozen oocytes for later use, but both methods are still experimental.

Autografting
Thawed slices of ovary might be grafted to the host, either to the remaining ovarian site or to an ectopic site such as the uterus or under the skin. With this technique, live births have been achieved in marmosets, sheep, mice, and recently in monkeys. To date, the only publicised attempt at human ovarian autotransplantation after cryopreservation was unsuccessful because folliculogenesis returned only for a short time. Indeed, preliminary experiments show that few oocytes survive in the tissue after grafting—sometimes the stored tissue is from patients with haematological or other malignancies with a propensity to metastasise, and so the safety of regrafting has been questioned.

In vitro maturation
Finding a reliable protocol for the in vitro maturation of immature follicles is a major challenge. Complete in vitro

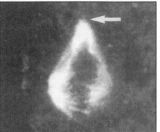

During cooling of an oocyte for cryopreservation, the normal metaphase spindle (left) can become dismantled (right), which could result in the production after fertilisation of a karyotypically abnormal embryo

A major challenge in the cryopreservation of oocytes is to (a) preserve the egg's ability to be fertilised and (b) maintain the integrity of its genetic material so that a genetically normal embryo is produced

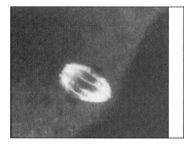

Live births after egg freezing are rare and can make headline news

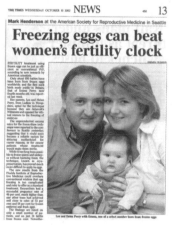

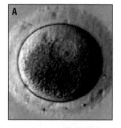

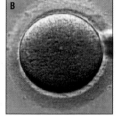

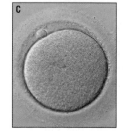

In in vitro maturation the germinal vesicle (within granular cytoplasm) of the immature oocyte (A) breaks down and the oocyte grows into a metaphase I oocyte (B). The egg becomes fully mature (metaphase II) when a polar body is extruded (C)

development of immature follicles has been achieved in mice, but culture of ovarian tissue from large mammals and humans is difficult because normal oocyte growth is often compromised. The current dilemma is whether young women undergoing chemical or surgical oophorectomy should take the precaution of having some ovarian tissue frozen. Only if today's cryopreservation techniques are appropriate would they be able to use the stored tissue in future for in vitro maturation (when these methods are developed).

Preserving fertility in prepubertal boys

Testicular tissue from prepubertal boys (before Tanner stage 2) does not contain mature spermatozoa and so cannot be used for assisted reproductive techniques without maturation in vitro. As it is not possible to collect an ejaculated sample, cryopreservation of surgically retrieved testicular tissue may be the only option. Besides the practical difficulties yet to be overcome in the use of immature sperm, retrieval of such tissue presents legal and ethical dilemmas because the child is unlikely to be old enough to give informed consent. The Royal College of Obstetricians and Gynaecologists and the British Fertility Society have produced guidelines for storage and use.

Preimplantation genetic diagnosis

Preimplantation genetic diagnosis (PGD) is an early alternative to prenatal diagnosis and is suitable for patients who are at substantial risk of conceiving a pregnancy affected by a known genetic defect. The technique has been applied to the analysis of numerical and structural chromosomal abnormalities that can result in handicap or recurrent miscarriage, the identification of sex to prevent transmission of X linked disease, and for the detection of specific serious monogenic disorders.

For PGD, one or two cells are removed from embryos at the early cleavage stage and the diagnostic test is carried out on these cells. The genetic status of the embryo is inferred from the result of the test, and only unaffected embryos are placed in the uterus. For single gene disorders, such as cystic fibrosis and spinal muscular atrophy, the polymerase chain reaction is used to amplify the region of the DNA containing the genetic lesion to levels where a diagnostic test can be carried out.

PGD of sex linked diseases for which the specific genetic defect is unknown or not amenable to molecular diagnosis at the single cell level can be done using fluorescence in situ hybridisation (FISH). Probes that bind to specific chromosomal telomeres can be used to identify balanced or unbalanced products in Robertsonian and reciprocal translocations.

PGD is a highly specialised procedure that is available at only a few reproductive medicine centres worldwide, and the number of live births achieved is still relatively small. However, the use of this technique will expand rapidly as the molecular basis for more diseases is found.

Preimplantation screening of embryos

Implanting multiple embryos has led to an unacceptably high rate of multiple births. As the aim of assisted conception is to produce a healthy baby, reducing multiple pregnancy rates is a major goal and transferring a single embryo is the ideal. The ability to identify embryos with high implantation potential will allow more effective selection of embryos for embryo transfer and reduce the likelihood of multiple pregnancy without reducing overall pregnancy rates.

Preserving men's fertility
- Testicular function is often compromised after chemotherapy treatment in much the same way as described above for ovarian tissue
- Preservation of fertility for men is much more straightforward than for women
- Freezing of multiple samples of ejaculated semen before chemotherapy and radiotherapy is successful
- Men about to have chemotherapy should be offered cryostorage of sperm as good practice

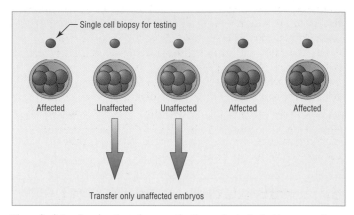

The principle of preimplantation genetic diagnosis. A single blastomere is removed from each 8-cell human embryo for the purposes of preimplantation genetic diagnosis. Up to two embryos found to be unaffected by the genetic disorder are transferred to the uterus

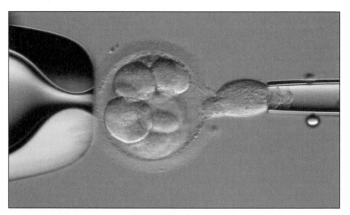

A single cell being removed from an 8-cell human embryo in vitro for genetic testing

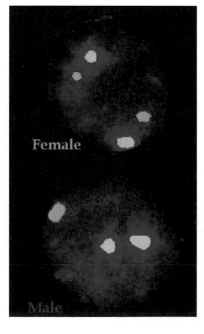

Preimplantation diagnosis using fluorescence in situ hybridisation (FISH). Specific probes, which bind to either X (green) or Y (red) chromosomes in the interphase nucleus fluoresce under ultraviolet illumination are used to determine the sex of the embryo

Selection of embryos for transfer is generally made on morphological grounds. Early cleavage stage embryos graded as high quality seem to have an improved implantation potential, although specificity is poor.

Some women, including those in older age groups (>38 years) and those who have had repeated failure of in vitro fertilisation, are more likely to produce cytogenetically abnormal embryos, which are not capable of normal development. For these patients, preimplantation genetic screening or aneuploidy screening has been advocated. By using techniques developed for PGD to select normal embryos, the chromosomes that are responsible for the major survivable aneuploidies (for example, 21, 22, 18, 13, X, and Y) can be examined from an embryo biopsy using fluorescence in situ hybridisation. As over half of all embryos can be cytogenetically abnormal, excluding these embryos from selection has improved ongoing implantation rates in some studies. However, the restriction to the common aneuploidies still allows those embryos that may have other chromosomal rearrangements to remain undetected. This limits the usefulness of the screening.

Stem cells and therapeutic cloning

Much media hype has surrounded the prospects of using embryonic stem cells in the treatment of degenerative diseases and the in vivo repair of damaged tissues. Potential treatments range from restoration of spinal cord function after injury to the cure of diabetes by replenishment of insulin producing cells of the pancreas. Neurological, hepatic, and cardiac or skeletal muscle cell lines derived from mouse embryos have all been used successfully in several mouse model systems to ameliorate symptoms previously untreatable by conventional treatment. However, derivation of embryonic stem cell lines in humans is more difficult. Many problems still have to be overcome before there is any prospect of their use in treatment.

In the United Kingdom, after heated debate in both Houses and following the advice of a select committee of the House of Lords, legislation has been passed that allows research using human stem cells derived from human embryos that are surplus to in vitro fertilisation programmes. Creation of stem cell lines tailored to be immunologically compatible by cell nuclear replacement (therapeutic cloning) is also permitted, as is the creation of embryos specifically for this purpose. However, creation and use of human embryos in vitro falls under the Human Fertilisation and Embryology Act, and the Human Fertilisation and Embryology Authority (HFEA) will examine all requests. It is a requirement of an HFEA licence that a sample of the line is lodged with the newly created stem cell bank of the Medical Research Council, which will administer the use of the deposited cell lines by third parties.

Competing interests: None declared.

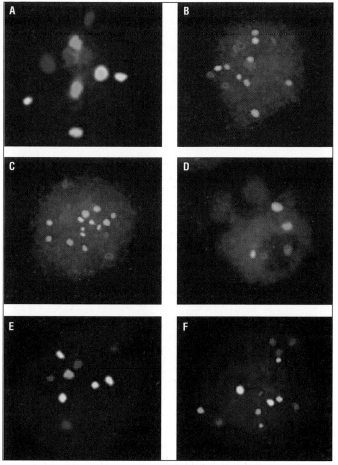

Aneuploidy screening—normal embryos are diploid and have two spots for each colour (A). Many different abnormalities have been seen; some are shown above. The complete set of chromosomes has been duplicated in triploid (B) and tetraploid (C) nuclei. A set of chromosomes is missing in haploid embryos (D). Abnormalities of individual chromosomes are also seen (E), such as monosomy, trisomy, and double trisomy (F). If embryos with such abnormalities could be screened out, a higher implantation rate might be achieved after in vitro fertilisation

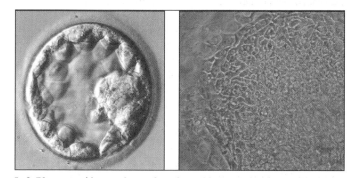

Left: Blastocyst with outer layer of trophectoderm and clear inner cell mass. Right: Human embryonic stem cells derived originally from the inner cell mass

---

Further reading

- Chief Medical Officer's Expert Group on Therapeutic Cloning. Stem cells: medical progress with responsibility. DoH, 2000 www.doh.gov.uk/cegc/stemcellreport.htm
- Stem cell research report of House of Lords select committee. Stationery Office, 2002 www.publications.parliament.uk/pa/ld/ldstem.htm
- Royal College of Obstetricians and Gynaecologists Working Party. *Storage of ovarian and prepubertal testicular tissue.* London: RCOG, 2000
- Multidisciplinary Working Group of the British Fertility Society. A strategy for fertility services for survivors of childhood cancer. *Hum Fertil* 2003;6:1-40
- Braude P, Pickering S, Flinter F, Mackie Ogilvie C. Preimplantation genetic diagnosis. *Nat Gen Rev* 2002:3:941-53
- Flinter F. Preimplantation diagnosis. *BMJ* 2001;322:1008-9
- Department of Health. *Preimplantation genetic diagnosis (PGD)—guiding principles for commissioners of NHS services.* London: DoH, 2002

Index

Page numbers in **bold** denote figures, those in *italics* refer to tables/boxed material.

Index

The complete ABC series

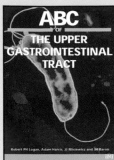
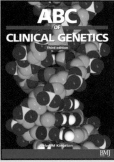
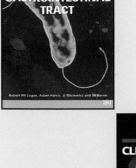
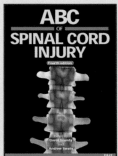
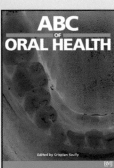
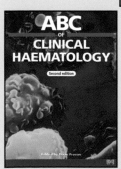